Delivered From ADHD

Overcoming ADHD in Adults and Children

By

Tirath S Gill MD

Prof. Paramjeet Singh MD

Contributions by

Sahiba Singh MD

Shaleen Gill MD

Dedication

To
Individuals
With
ADHD
&
ADD

Contents

Disclaimer

No book can replace the services of a qualified health professional. Please use this book to help you communicate more effectively with your doctor so that you can obtain the best possible care. This book is not intended as a guide for self-medication. Treatment of ADHD and other psychiatric conditions should be delivered by a qualified health care professional in the context of a patient doctor relationship. The author and publisher expressly disclaim responsibility for any negative effects directly or indirectly attributable to the use or application of any information contained in this book.

Acknowledgements

We thank the patients and their families that we have had the privilege of working with. They have helped us understand the real life difficulties and complications related to ADHD. This would be most difficult to grasp merely through the pages of any book alone. This book is dedicated to these patients with ADHD that work to overcome their difficulties.

Ms. Michelle Owhadi and Mr. Paul Owhadi of the California Psychological Institute (CPI) have been exemplary in creating a supportive climate for clinicians and case managers that work with foster children and foster families. CPI over the years has been able to help many disenfranchised children and families of Fresno County and the surrounding areas. The many fine clinicians, therapists and case managers that work here are also acknowledged. They are making a real difference for the better in this world.

Ms. Diane Rose, Christie Henry, Mayra Aguirre, Beatriz Sanchez, and others from Adventist Hospital are also appreciated for their tireless efforts. They have done much in getting psychiatric services for residents in the small townships of the central valley such as Selma and Hanford. Lastly, we are most grateful to many colleagues and friends at SMS Medical College Jaipur, and at the Fresno VA Hospital for sharing their insights and experience. They have validated the idea in a resounding manner that the treatment of ADHD is a worthwhile endeavor.

Tirath S Gill MD   Prof. Paramjeet Singh MD

Tirath Gill finished his residency at Yale Psychiatry Program. He has been board certified in General Psychiatry, Forensic Psychiatry, Addiction Psychiatry and Psychosomatic Medicine. He is currently a Chief Psychiatrist for the California Department of Corrections and Rehabilitation.

Professor Paramjeet Singh is a professor of psychiatry at SMS Singh Medical College in Jaipur India. He has published in several peer reviewed journals. He is also active in the psychiatry residency training program. He is an advocate for universal healthcare and for making psychiatric services available for individuals in the underserved areas.

Preface

A diffuse and multifaceted syndrome of inattention and impulsivity called ADHD is more prevalent than you would think. The acronym ADHD stands for Attention Deficit Hyperactivity Disorder. It is a relatively common clinical condition but is often not recognized. The dysfunction caused by it is attributed to other factors. ADD (Attention Deficit disorder) is another name this condition goes by and is essentially the same syndrome of ADHD without the hyperactivity component. The H of ADHD denoting hyperactivity is taken out of the acronym to get ADD.

For the purposes of discussion in this book, the term ADHD subsumes the diagnosis of both ADD and ADHD.

There are a great many studies on this subject. When all the studies are put together, they indicate prevalence for ADHD of about 6 percent in children and about 3 to 4 percent in adults. The national comorbidity survey actually indicates a prevalence of 4.4 percent in adults but we have downplayed this figure. This still represents a large number of children and adults that could be impaired by ADHD. They could stand to benefit from proper recognition and treatment when symptoms cause problems in their lives.

This book looks at the various aspects of ADHD and provides education about the symptoms and the different treatment options. We have resorted to a question and answer format in some sections. In other areas, diagrams and tables are provided to make the book more user friendly. The questions may sometimes sound repetitive but the answers may reveal a different aspect of the same issue.

Experience indicates that for mild degrees of ADHD, nonpharmacological interventions (treatment without medications) may suffice. When problems caused by ADHD cause significant dysfunction, medications may be safely used to bring about relief. Medications are used in conjunction with the nonpharmacological measures.

These measures are beneficial in a great majority of patients diagnosed with ADHD.

As in the treatment of other psychiatric conditions, the benefit and risks of any medications used should be carefully considered. In order to increase the level of safety with medications for ADHD, it is important for the clinician to get a detailed history of any medical issues, cardiovascular problems, or fainting spells in the past. He or she may also enquire if there is a history of sudden death at a young age in the family. Such events in other family members may indicate some inherited medical issues that can increase the risk for adverse events.

Some patients and their family members may have concerns about the dependence and abuse risk of stimulant drugs used to treat ADHD. The risk for this is low in the properly diagnosed ADHD patient but not insignificant. If there is a history of substance abuse problems in the past, the use of stimulants should be avoided. For them, nonstimulant medications are available and may offer a better treatment option. The patient and family members should feel free to discuss any medication anxieties or concerns with the treating doctor.

This book attempts to address educational needs and interests of three types of readers- the person diagnosed with ADHD, the concerned family member and the treating clinicians. The section on pharmacological treatments is mostly geared for clinicians with background in pharmacology. It may be too technical for the average reader. An effort has been made to keep the jargon out. This is more difficult than we had at first realized.

Any medication trial should be initiated only by a physician or a clinician licensed to prescribe who is familiar with the risks and benefits of the medications. The doctor will watch for symptom improvement and monitor for any side effects. The common side effects and strategies for managing them are also discussed in this book.

The treatments discussed are those that have been used successfully in our own practice and by many others. Real world experience is always a little different from the ivory tower notions. We have advocated a conservative approach of going low and going slow with any medication in order to avoid side effects.

This book also does not need to be read cover to cover to derive benefits. There may be some overlap in the content at times when it is relevant to repeat an idea.

Although efforts have been made to assure accuracy of factual data in reference to medications, some inaccuracies may have crept in during the publication process. The reader is advised to always check with other standard references to confirm dosages etc.

When ADHD patients are properly diagnosed and offered a balanced treatment plan; they are able to achieve the level of success that was elusive in the past. Their efforts that were dispersed in many directions previously can finally be harnessed and focused on the issues pertinent to their lives. The benefits can at times be dramatic.

Please enjoy the book and use whatever makes sense to you. One does not have to use all the techniques that are discussed to derive some benefit. Some of the information on nonpharmacological interventions may be helpful in improving focus even if you do not suffer from ADHD.

This book is organized into the following sections: A history of ADHD, followed by a discussion of the different symptoms. This is followed by a special chapter on ADHD affecting adults, which is then followed by a discussion of the different treatment options. Some important medical conditions that may present with problems of inattention are discussed followed by some miscellaneous topics and resources for further reading and help. The pronoun he may be used in some sections of the book for convenience. The discussion of issues related to ADHD however is equally relevant to both the genders.

The broad outline of this book is depicted in the following diagram.

Chapter 1
A Brief History of ADHD

"It isn't the mountains ahead that wear you out; it's the grain of sand in your shoes." Anonymous

A distinct clinical condition resembling ADHD was recognized by Hippocrates over 2000 years ago. He opined as depicted in the below diagram that some individuals have quickened responses implying impulsivity and less tenaciousness indicating a high level of distractibility.

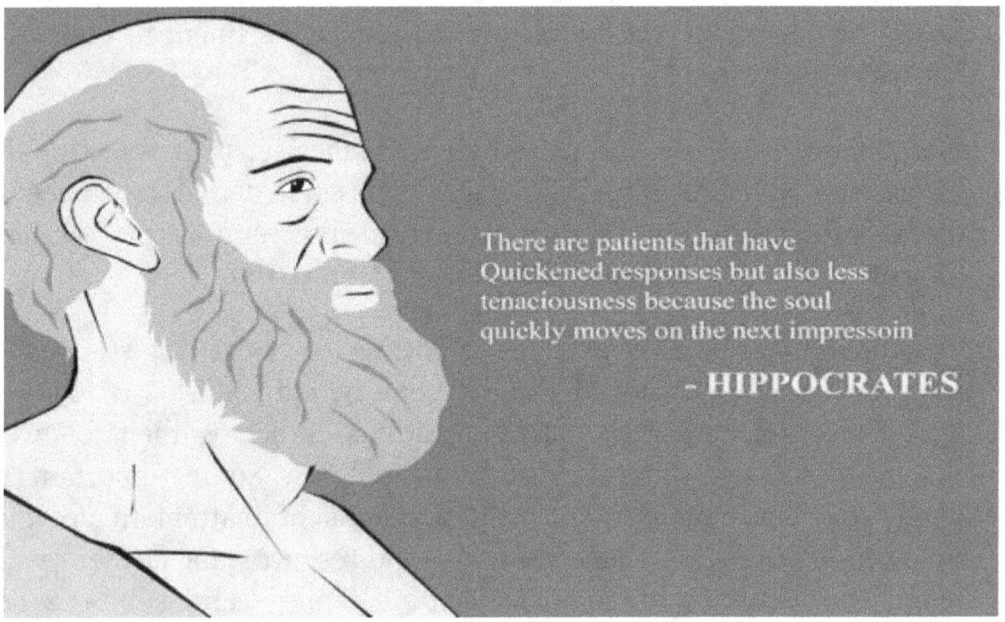

There are patients that have Quickened responses but also less tenaciousness because the soul quickly moves on the next impressoin

- HIPPOCRATES

He seems to be describing a clinical condition that fits the clinical picture of ADHD. Hippocrates attributed this condition to an "overbalance of fire over water."

He reasoned according to the four-humor theory of the time that an excess of "fire" caused some folks to be hyperactive and to have an excitable temperament.

Here is a little background on Hippocrates. He lived in ancient Greece around 500 BC and is best known for asking his students to follow certain moral principles. Nowadays, these principles are codified and known as the Hippocratic Oath. This oath is taken by graduating doctors around the world and forms the bedrock of medical ethics.

It enjoins and asks all physicians to first do no harm to their patients and to always advocate for their welfare. For his high moral standards and for his love of teaching medicine, Hippocrates has been rightly crowned as the Father of Medicine. He is famous for advocating the use of logic to deduce the nature of the problem from the given facts and for devising logical solutions to the problems the patient faced.

After this ray of insight, for the next two millennia the syndrome of inattention and impulsivity did not garner much thought or comment. Then, in the year 1845, Dr. Heinrich Hoffman wrote about a condition in a fictional character called Fidgety Phil that enumerated almost all the symptoms found in children with ADHD.

About 50 years later, in 1902, Dr. George F. Still observed ADHD related symptoms in a group of children that were under his care. He reported that these children were unique due to their heightened impulsivity and behavioral problems. According to Still, these symptoms were caused by a genetic dysfunction and not by poor parenting.

He elaborated on this finding through lectures to the Royal College of Physicians in London. These were called the "Goulstonian lectures" and he talked more about these kids. The name of his lecture is alluring and invited much interest. The title was 'Some Abnormal Psychical Conditions in Children'.

These children were described by him as often aggressive, defiant, and resistant to discipline. They were also noted to be excessively emotional or "passionate". His comments on heightened impulsivity were insightful as he remarked that they showed "little inhibitory volition, and could not learn from the consequences of their actions, though their intellect was normal."

He opined in the concepts of those days, accordingly, "I would point out that a notable feature in many of these cases of moral defect without general impairment of intellect is a quite abnormal incapacity for sustained attention".

He went on to write an article that was published later in the well-regarded journal Lancet. In his papers, he described 43 children who had serious problems with sustained attention and self-regulation.

In the year 1937, Dr. Charles Bradley administered Benzedrine. This was a medication with stimulant properties and was used at the time for the treatment of musculoskeletal aches. Dr. Bradley found to his surprise that Benzedrine also helped with hyperactivity and impulsivity in some of these children. He remarked and wrote about his findings but his observations were mostly forgotten.

Then, based on his finding, in 1956, another stimulant methylphenidate (Ritalin) was offered to children by some physicians for symptoms of hyperactivity. The benefits were remarkable and noticed by every clinician, parent, and teacher that was involved in these initial trials.

In the ensuing decade of the 1960's, the treatment of ADHD with stimulant medications became better recognized and more widely accepted. Interest from medical professionals increased in this condition and some landmark papers were written in the subsequent years. Some of these papers are as follows:

1. Menkes, Rowe and Menkes 1967 looked at childhood ADHD

2. Quitkin and Klein in 1969 described symptoms of ADHD in adults

It came to light that these children had higher than normal rates of difficult childbirth or of their mother having endured a complicated pregnancy. In such cases, the stress or "insult" to the developing brain was felt to be related the manifestation of ADHD later in their childhood. The hyperactivity was linked to some minimal brain damage (MBD) induced by these events. ADHD was for some time therefore also known as minimal brain damage syndrome and minimal brain disorder by others and referred to with the same acronym.

We currently do not use the term MBD to describe ADHD as there is no clear proof of brain damage in many cases. The fact remains true however that there are indications of altered brain functioning and a higher rate of stressful events in the early history of the individuals with ADHD.

It must be noted that in the 1970's, ADD came to be better recognized as a distinct syndrome of inattention without the hyperactivity. Many adults describe themselves to have ADD and not ADHD. Semantics aside, the treatments are similar as is the underlying pathophysiology.

Prospective long-term studies such as the Milwaukee study followed children diagnosed with ADHD into their adulthood. Based on the findings, it was recognized that ADHD does not always go into full remission by late adolescence but continues to be a problem in a residual form in adulthood for about 30 to 50 percent of the children with ADHD.

This works out to about 2 to 3 percent of the adults in the general population. This is a large number. Some unrecognized ADHD patients learn creative ways of overcoming their deficits. Others by trial and error learn to take up jobs where the ADHD works to their advantage.

For others, it continues to hamstring their social and occupational roles in different ways.

In 1994; a best-selling book titled "Driven to Distraction" was published. The authors Edward Hallowell and John Ratey were physicians who had struggled due to ADHD through their training at Harvard Medical School. In eloquent prose, they acquainted the public again with a condition that had slipped into oblivion.

Further changes have occurred in the new diagnostic manual DSM V. It has made provisions for the recognition of adult ADHD without the official diagnosis of ADHD in childhood or adolescence. This is reasonable since childhood ADHD is often not recognized or treated and documentation does not always exist for the presence of ADHD in childhood.

When it comes to treatment, for the most part, pharmacological treatment (treatment with medications) has been the main treatment approach. In the future however non-pharmacological treatments such as biofeedback and neurofeedback may play a greater role in offering relief from ADHD. There is a growing database on the usefulness and effectiveness of nonpharmacological interventions.

You may be wondering how this recount of history is relevant. We took the trouble to document this so as to show that the ADHD syndrome is real and not a hypothetical conjecture or a misperception. It is not something cooked up by drug companies to "sell their drugs".

It is a real condition with consequences for the person that suffers from it. With treatment, it can get better!

PROMINENT PEOPLE WITH ADHD

The following individuals have acknowledged that they have ADHD. They have reached heights of success despite their handicap and some would argue because of it. They have managed by sheer will to persevere in the face of all obstacles and adapt themselves to the liabilities imposed by their condition. They have all managed to reach a high level of success in their respective fields. This serves to underscore a point that individuals with ADHD sometimes have unique ways of thinking. They can come up with creative ideas and novel solutions for problems that may have vexed others. By their accomplishments, they serve as a beacon to greatness for others who may suffer from ADHD.

Michael Jordan

Michael Jordan is counted as one of the greatest basketball players of all time. It wasn't always the case however. Most people don't know that Jordan had to struggle with ADHD all through his schooling and college years. He achieved success by working hard and practicing more than his peers. To illustrate his perseverance despite the obstacles, he is known to have said the following.

"I've missed more than 9000 shots in my career. I've lost almost 300 games. 26 times, I've been trusted to take the game winning shot and missed. I've failed over and over and over again in my life. And that is why I succeed."

Michael Jordan is a great role model for anyone who struggles with their ADD or ADHD. They know by his example that a will to succeed and perseverance will overcome all obstacles that stand between them and their success.

RICHARD BRANSON

Knighted for his achievements and contributions to society, Richard Branson is one of the more well-known persons with ADHD. He has achieved great success with business enterprises such as Virgin Atlantic Airlines, Virgin Records and many other companies. His zeal and enthusiasm is undimmed by age and he is now planning in collaboration with others in the launching of a space tourism enterprise called Virgin Galactic. It is notable that he has achieved his success by recognizing his deficits, and strengths and building a great team that compliments each other. His success is attributable to his ability to inspire, and his belief in his own goals.

Branson has talked about how he made ADHD "work" for him, by believing his "crazy" dreams, instead of attempting to abide by advisors and friends that told him something could not be done.

Some other well-known people with ADD or ADHD are as follows:

Will Smith – A gifted actor, singer and humanitarian.

Jim Carrey- Famous actor who excels in slapstick comedy and parody roles in films.

Terry Bradshaw- Currently a sportscaster and a former hall of fame quarterback - the Pittsburgh Steelers. He took them to four super bowl championships.

James Carville – Political consultant and advocate; legendary campaign manager for President Bill Clinton

Paul Orfalea's -Successful Businessman, started the Kinkos office chain

David Neeleman – Founder of JetBlue Airways

Chapter 2
Defining ADHD

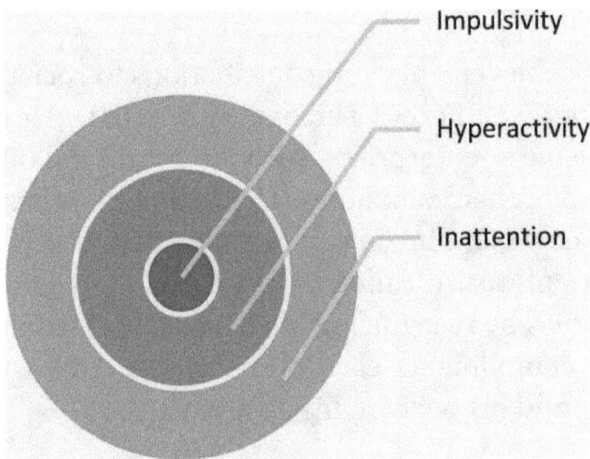

The core features of ADHD are hyperactivity, increased impulsivity, and inattention. In ADD, the inattentive component is more predominant and hyperactivity is less of an issue.

ADHD and ADD affects the day to day functioning of an individual. It is a diagnosis of exclusion after other causes of such symptoms have been ruled out. The diagnosis is not made lightly and it is not diagnosed if it is related to a medical condition, a substance induced intoxication or withdrawal from a substance. It is also not diagnosed if the distraction and inattention is due to emotional distress.

ADHD is classified as a neurodevelopmental disorder. This implies that there is a difference in the way that the ADHD brain develops; it is different from most other brains. The symptoms of ADHD are noticeable in early childhood and evident by the time the child is 7 years old. These symptoms are discussed later.

The cause of the syndrome of ADHD has been linked to an abnormal functioning in the frontal lobes. The frontal lobes are situated behind the forehead and function as finely tuned brakes for the rest of the nervous system. When their functioning is impaired, the net result is state of motor hyperactivity along with a tendency to be easily distracted. Poor impulse control is another notable feature. This is schematically represented in the following diagram.

Frontal Lobe Functions

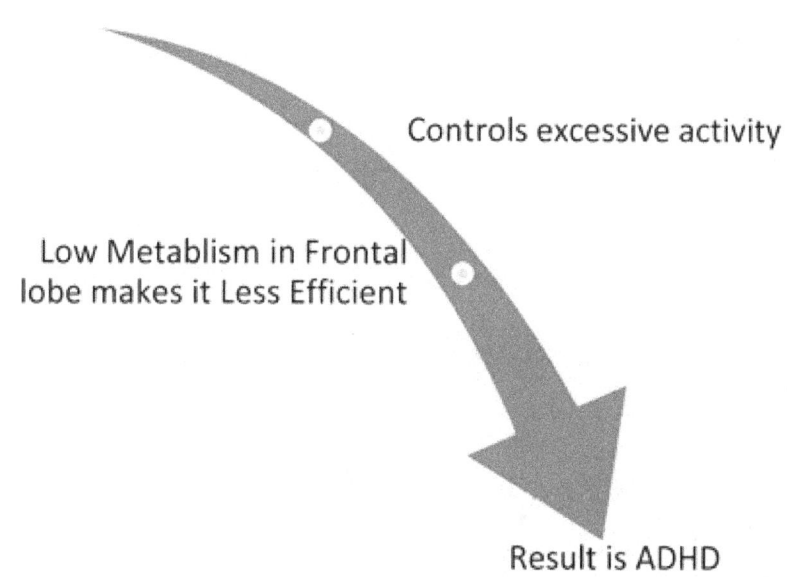

Controls excessive activity

Low Metablism in Frontal lobe makes it Less Efficient

Result is ADHD

First Manifestations of ADHD:

The child shows symptoms of hyperactivity, inattention and impulsivity. First time parents often notice the hyperactivity but ascribe it to normal childhood behaviors. It is only after repeated complaints from the teachers that they may seek consultation.

The Three Types of ADHD

Current nomenclature classifies ADHD into three subtypes depending on the predominance of either hyperactivity or inattention. The three types of ADHD based on this scheme are as follows:

1. **ADHD, Combined Type**: In this, there is an almost equal mixture of all the symptoms of hyperactivity, impulsivity and inattention. This is the most common pattern.

2. **ADHD, Predominantly Inattentive Type**: This is also called ADD. In this type, the hyperactive symptoms are not as prominent and the symptoms of inattention and daydreaming predominate.

3. **ADHD, Predominantly Hyperactive-Impulsive Type**: In this type, impulsive and aggressive intrusive behaviors are the predominant feature.

EVIDENCE FOR ADHD AS A STATE OF ALTERED METABOLISM

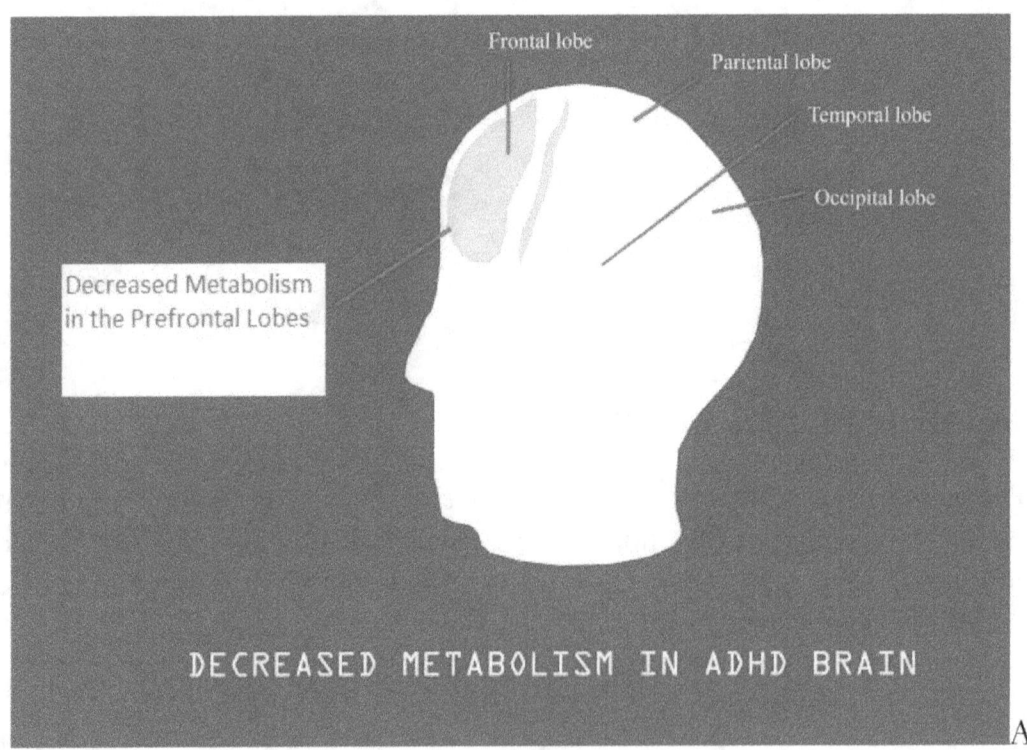

16

A state of lowered metabolism in the frontal lobes of ADHD brains has been noted. The basis for the above is a pioneering neuroimaging study done in 1990 by Zametken and colleagues.

Zametkin, A. J., Nordahl, T. E., Gross, M., King, A. C., Semple, W. E., Rumsey, J., Hamburger, S., & Cohen, R. M. (1990). Cerebral glucose metabolism in adults with hyperactivity of childhood onset. *New England Journal of Medicine, 323,* 1361-1366.

They used PET scans (positron emission tomography scans) to measure glucose metabolism in the brain of 25 adults with ADHD symptoms. They compared these with 25 control patients who did not have ADHD. They found a lowered state of metabolism in the prefrontal lobes as depicted in the above diagram.

These PET scans indicated decreased frontal lobe functioning. This is felt to be related to a decrease in the ability to sustain focus and attention and increased impulsivity and activity in these individuals.

A LIST OF ADHD SYMPTOMS

(Source ICD and DSM V - ICD=International Classification of Diseases; DSM= Diagnostic and Statistical Manual of Mental Disorders)

The symptoms are as follows:

Symptoms of Inattention Spectrum:

1. Being forgetful in daily activities. This may involve forgetting appointments or objects such as books, keys, purse, etc.

2. Being late for appointments due to procrastination.

3. Being easily distracted by other stimuli in the environment

4. Perpetual disorganization of desk and workspace

5. Poor organization and planning

6. Inability to finish tasks on time or to finish them at all

7. Difficulty in following directions

8. Procrastination and putting things off till the last minute.

9. Appearing lost, distracted, and confused when spoken to

10. The individual has lapses of attention and may ask to repeat things that were told to him or her earlier.

11. Forgetting the original train of thought and having to reread the same information again

12. Glossing over details and making careless mistakes

13. Being annoyed by tasks that require sustained attention such as game of chess.

Symptoms of hyperactivity and impulsivity spectrum

1. Fidgeting, squirming, moving out of the chair when expected to sit still

2. In adults, it may manifest as emotional impulsivity

3. It may also be noticeable by an inability to sit through meetings

4. The person may experience a sense of internal restlessness

5. Excessive running around, climbing on furniture

6. Engaging in risky play activity that may result in accidents and injury

7. ADHD child may seem constantly moving "as if driven by a motor" and "always on the go".

8. In adulthood, it may involve working on multiple projects at the same time.

9. The child may create a lot of noise and clutter during play activities.

10. In the adult, their living and work environment may be disorganized and messy.

11. Excessive talking, blurting out answers. This may continue into adulthood and involve activities such as finishing sentences for others.

12. Impulsive decision making

13. Disruptive and intrusive behaviors.

14. Violation of rules and social norms such as speeding, getting into altercations.

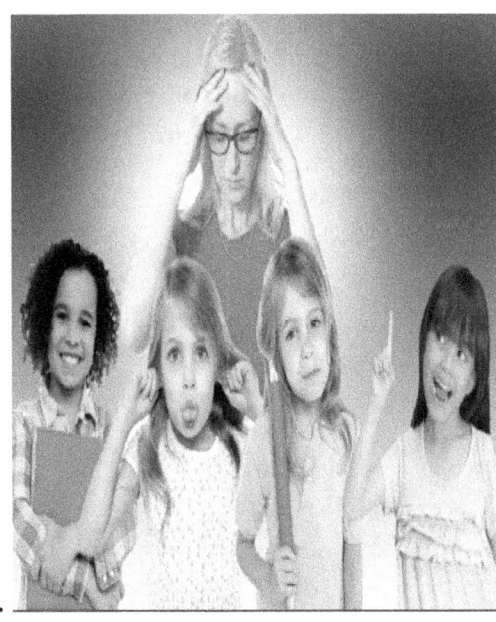

Children with ADHD can be disruptive and difficult for the teacher to manage.

Teacher Rating Scales for ADHD are useful for assessment and monitoring.

15.

The Hyperactive Child – A Diagram

ADHD

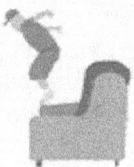

ADHD is a condition marked by 6 or more symptoms of hyperactivity, impulsivity or inattention. These symptoms lead to dysfunction in two or more settings in the individual's life.

HYPERACTIVITY SYMPTOMS

Always on the go, excessive running, squirming, moving around, loud disorganized play, excessive talking, blurting our answers, difficulty waiting for turn, impulsive decision making, rash behaviors, disruptive and intrusive behaviors

Leaves seat when remaining seated is required, fidgets with hand and feet excessive motor activity continues at different locations, unable to modulate behaviors

INATTENTION SYMPTOMS

Forgetfulness, not turning homework in, losing objects, forgetting lunch, unfinished tasks, difficulty folowing directions, missing appointments, daydreaming, difficulty with details, making careless mistakes, easily distracted, appears unfocussed when spoken to.

The diagnostic criteria of ADHD state that if there are 6 or more symptoms related to ADHD in two or more settings and if these symptoms cause dysfunction for a period of 6 or more months, the person may have ADHD.

Before a diagnosis of ADHD is made, the complete biopsychosocial context of the behaviors including any medical and emotional causes should be considered..

For a diagnosis of ADHD or ADD in adults, it is a requirement that there be documentation of ADHD in childhood of the person. As many adults with ADHD may not have documentation of childhood symptoms, this criterion has been revised in the DSM V to allow for an exception to a childhood diagnosis. If it can be shown by other collateral information that a dysfunction in childhood existed, a diagnosis of adult ADHD can be made.

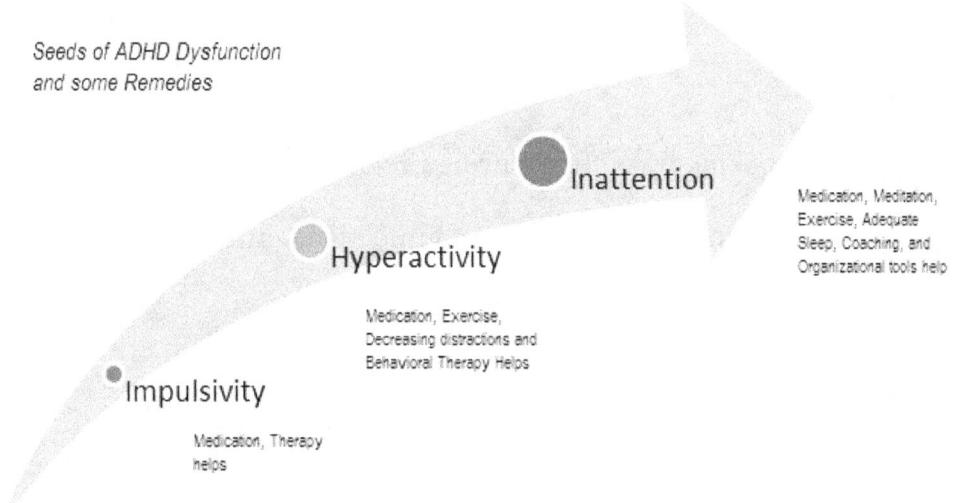

Seeds of ADHD Dysfunction and some Remedies

Inattention
Medication, Meditation, Exercise, Adequate Sleep, Coaching, and Organizational tools help

Hyperactivity
Medication, Exercise, Decreasing distractions and Behavioral Therapy Helps

Impulsivity
Medication, Therapy helps

Normal Brain Development

The development of the brain is not complete at birth. Brain growth and development continues from the embryonic stage to age 21 as countless nerve cells (neurons) migrate and establish contacts with one another. They interact in complex ways in a finely orchestrated manner. An alteration may occur due to infections during pregnancy of the mother or in young childhood or due any number of other causes listed later. In fact, environment plays an important role and no two brain developments are always alike. There may be differences even among identical twins if they grow up in different environments. A slight change in brain development can lead to dysfunction that can becomes evident as ADHD. The dysfunction may also become evident as a learning disorder or a form of autism called pervasive developmental disorder. ADHD is one such product of the interaction of environment and the genetics of the developing brain.

Individuals with ADHD can be of subnormal, normal or high intelligence.

Risk Factors

Some of the following risk factors have been associated with ADHD.

1. Poor nutrition

2. Cigarette smoking by mother during pregnancy,

3. Alcohol, substance abuse issues, and infections during the pregnancy

4. Difficult labor

5. Genetics

WHO IS USUALLY THE FIRST TO RECOGNIZE ADHD?

The teacher in kindergarten or early primary school is often the first to notice a problem. Most teachers are educated about ADHD and are able to recognize the problem in their pupils.

To the parent, the teacher may report behavioral problems in the child. This may include difficulty in following rules or it may involve intrusive and disruptive behaviors with other students in the classroom. They may report that the child is unable to remain in his assigned seat or is noted to push or pull on other children.

RECOGNITION OF ADHD IN ADULTS

Recognition in adults often comes about in a roundabout way. An adult may read about ADHD and subsequently present themselves to a doctor for an evaluation. Most adults that have the condition are usually correct about their hunch. Caution does not need to be exercised however as some symptoms of inattention or forgetfulness are universal at some time or another. It is only the persistent nature of ADHD symptoms that warrants a diagnosis and treatment consideration.

CONSEQUENCES OF UNTREATED ADHD

ADHD *can* be an obstacle to finishing projects and achieving goals. This can lead academic and occupational underachievement. The affected person may not realize that they have ADHD. Some consequences of untreated ADHD are benign while others are more serious.

Below are some of the consequences of untreated ADHD.

Adverse or Negative Consequences of ADHD in Childhood

- Increased risk of not finishing school

- Higher risk for being suspended from school

- Higher risk for teenage pregnancy

- Higher risk for accidents in driving and in other activities

- Higher risk for experimentation with drugs and alcohol

- Higher risk of arrest for delinquent behaviors

- Higher risk for physical abuse, verbal abuse and neglect

Adverse or Negative Consequences of ADHD in Adulthood

- Increased risk for academic underachievement

- Increases risk for occupational underachievement

- Increases risk for divorce

- Increases risk for domestic violence

- Increases risk for arrest and incarceration

- Increases risk for being fired from the job and being unemployed

- Increases risk for substance and alcohol abuse

Benefits of knowing about ADHD

If you are knowledgeable about the signs, and symptoms of ADHD, you can recognize this problem in your child, spouse or even yourself. This may lead to a consultation with a doctor or a therapist that is skilled in the treatment of this condition. With the right treatment or combination of treatments, a dramatic improvement in functioning is possible.

WHAT PERCENTAGE OF ADHD CHILDREN HAVE LEARNING DISORDERS AS WELL?

It is estimated that 20 % or more of children that have ADHD issues may also have problems with other learning disorders. Such learning disorders may be developmental reading disorder, developmental mathematics disorder, or dyslexia.

HOW ARE ADHD BEHAVIORS DIFFERENT FROM NORMAL PLAYFULNESS IN A CHILD?

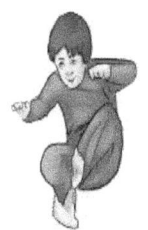

Many normal kids can be playful, rambunctious, inattentive and hyperactive at times.

The key difference however with ADHD kids is the degree and duration of the symptoms and the inability of the children to control themselves.

They can appear to almost be driven as if by a motor and have an inability to remain still or seated for any length of time. They continue to engage in these behaviors outside of playtimes.

The group behavior of rambunctious boys during some activities is unlikely to be sustained when playtime is over.

In contrast to this, the child with ADHD is unable to restrain or curb the hyperactivity, even when playtime is over. They are unable to comply when asked to be quiet in settings such as when at a church or when in a classroom. Their behavior seems beyond their control and they seem to almost be driven by a motor that will not let them stop.

The child also seems to recognize the problem but is unable to help themselves. They ask for something to help them "stay out of trouble" as their own efforts have often not been successful.

The following table summarizes some of the key points of difference between normal childhood playfulness and ADHD caused hyperactivity.

BEHAVIOR	NORMAL CHILD	CHILD WITH ADHD
Hyperactivity - Amenability to redirection	The hyperactivity is easily redirected by parent or teacher if it gets out of hand	The behavior is hard to redirect and may fail to improve with multiple reprimands and redirection
Duration	The playful hyperactive behavior is episodic and during play time or other limited periods	The hyperactive, distractible behavior tends to be more persistent and occurs in multiple settings. The child is unable to modulate this adequately unless keenly focused on an area of intense interest to them
Ability to rest calmly	Normal children are able to come to a point of relaxed, restful awareness	The ADHD child is unable to sit still and continues to fidget or move about as if driven by a motor
Ability to follow directions	Generally has an easier time of following directions correctly and more easily	May forget key parts of the directions or require multiple repetitions of directions. May continue to make mistakes in following directions.
Distractibility	Is able to ignore distracting stimuli more	Is more easily distracted by extraneous stimuli
BEHAVIOR Finishing tasks	NORMAL CHILD May need prompting but has a higher success rate in finishing tasks	ADHD CHILD Has more problems in finishing tasks such as homework or other assignments even with prompts and reminders. May forget to take homework to school.
Inattention	May have moments of inattention but is able to refocus	May be continuously unable to focus on the task at hand . May be prone to daydreaming.

Sleep difficulties	Unusual	May be noted

BEHAVIOR	NORMAL CHILD	CHILD WITH ADHD
Impulsivity	Is able to usually think of consequences before actions	May be prone to acting impulsively and rashly, resulting in greater incidence of accidents, conduct problems. There may be a higher incidence of unlawful behaviors in older ages due to impulsivity.
Difficulty with details	Is able to pay attention when needed to details	Has a great difficulty in tasks that require sustained attention and may gloss over details and directions leading to careless mistakes. These behaviors may continue into adulthood

PREVALENCE   OF
ADHD

The different surveys regarding the prevalence for ADHD indicate a mean prevalence of 5 to 6 percent in children. In adults, the prevalence rate is 3 to 4 percent of the adult population. The following bar chart breaks up the childhood prevalence into subcomponents of 2 percent in girls and 4 percent in boys. This is also supported by the demographic studies.

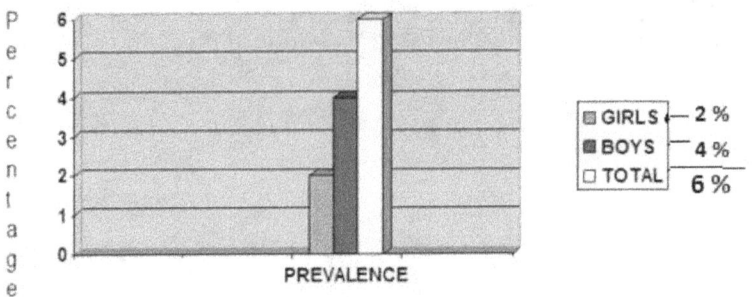

**THE PREVALENCE OF ADHD IN
BOYS AND GIRLS**

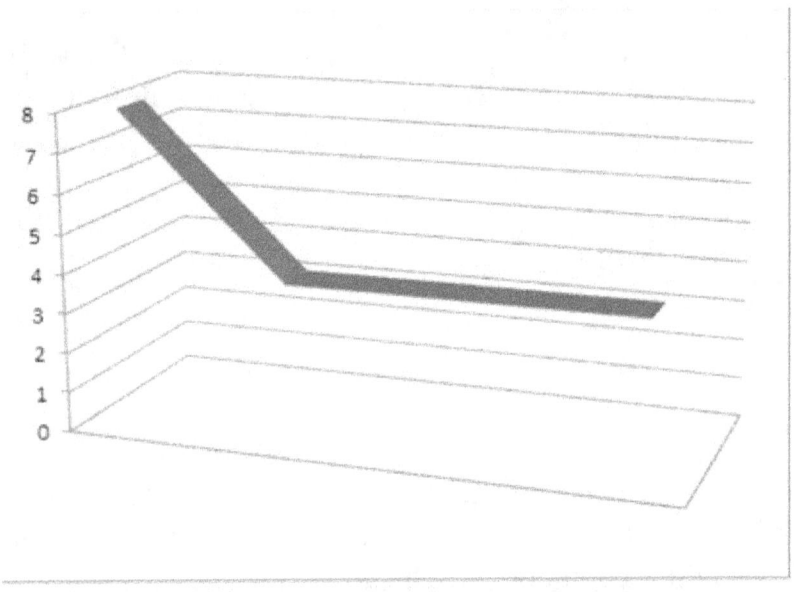

*The Declining Prevalence of ADHD
from Childhood to Adulthood*

With growth towards adulthood, the hyperactivity of ADHD decreases and is less noticeable in adults. The hyperactivity and impulsivity may take on new forms such as impulsive decision making and rash driving.

In adulthood, the ratio between men and women with ADHD is 1:1 with an equal number of women and men having ADHD. This is different from the 2:1 ratio seen between boys and girls.

PREPARING FOR AN ADHD CONSULT

1. Find Names of Doctors that Treat ADHD

One should first find out which doctors in the community treat ADHD as not every doctor is qualified to do so.

2. Find Names of Therapists that Treat ADHD

Look into therapists that treat ADHD as well if you want to explore treatment without medications.

3. Gather Report Cards:

Gather any school records indicating ADHD related behaviors such as inconsistent grades, teacher comments or reprimand notices for disruptive behaviors.

4. Take Collateral Sources

In the case of adults, it is useful to have a collateral source of information. This may be parents, a spouse or a colleague that knows the person well.

5. Take Results of Tests

Take any records of psychometric testing done such as intelligence tests.

Bring any rating scales such as a Conner's rating scale done by a teacher or other person that has the ability to observe the person over a period of time.

6. Gather Medical Records

Take along any medical records

Take a list of medications and over the counter supplements that may be taken.

Take along any recent laboratory test or EKG results if you have them

Pica is the eating of non- nutritional material such as clay, dirt, paint chips etc. If such behaviors exist, this should also be reported.

Any history of significant head injury should be reported.

7. Gather Information about Early Childhood

Be prepared to answer questions about early life development. This may include whether the person was full term or premature, of low birth weight or if there were any complications at childbirth.

There may be questions about any use of alcohol, tobacco or drugs by the mother during the pregnancy.

If there were any delays in beginning to sit (6 months), or stand and take first few steps (12 months) or talk, this should be shared with the doctor.

REACTION OF PATIENTS WHEN TOLD ABOUT ADHD

The parents of children with ADHD are often relieved when they hear that there is an explanation for the difficulties their child has been experiencing. Adults that receive the diagnosis in themselves may also experience similar relief. They are able to put their past difficulties in perspective. They recognize that their prior dysfunction was caused by a treatable condition and not a personal weakness of will or laziness.

A title of a popular book goes something like this- "You mean I am not lazy, stupid or crazy?" This statement underscores how patients of ADHD find relief when they hear the name of the condition that makes life difficult for them.

Recognition of ADHD and subsequent treatment helps to usher in a positive change in their life.

The understanding of the condition by the family also creates a more supportive environment for the person. Education of the family is therefore encouraged.

CAN THERE BE MORE THAN ONE REASON FOR DISORGANIZATION AND CLUTTER IN A PERSON'S LIFE?

Disorganization, hoarding and clutter can be due to a number of different causes. It can be a sign of unresolved conflicts, unresolved anxieties, incipient psychosis, dementia, depression or other conditions discussed later.

If it is determined that ADHD is the cause, medication along with cognitive behavioral therapy and teaching of organizational skills can make a significant difference. If the cause is due to a psychiatric disorder, appropriate treatments are often available for these conditions as well.

ADHD SYMPTOMS MAY EVOLVE AND CHANGE IN ADULTHOOD

The manifestations of ADHD change from childhood to adulthood. In childhood, the hyperactive symptoms predominate, especially in boys. As the child gets older, the hyperactive symptoms tend to decrease. The problems with inattention and distractibility may persist.

Hyperactivity in adults can present itself as a tendency for making decisions that are impulsive or rash without consideration of the consequences. Although, one can never make a perfect decision and consider every consequence, the normal person is able to weigh the obvious pro's and con's of any decision. The adult with ADHD may act on impulse and justify the decision later. Adult ADHD may also be colored by symptoms of anxiety, and a sense of unease.

EMOTIONAL COMPLICATIONS OF ADHD

The patient with ADHD may have social difficulties due to poor performance or underperformance. The individual may be typecast into a stereotype of being lazy, ne'er-do-well or a troublemaker. This mislabeling can create resentment, anxiety or depression in some individuals with ADHD.

Most people often do not understand the reason for the patient's difficulties. Sometimes the person with ADHD also does not understand the cause of their dysfunction and may blame himself or herself.

Dysphoria is a term used to describe a mixed state of unease and mild depression. In the absence of an understanding of the hidden problem of ADHD, the person may become dysphoric and perplexed. They know and recognize that they are capable of better things.

They may seek psychotherapy and counselling. Although such counselling may help with anxiety and depression, the underlying problem of ADHD is often not recognized. Much psychotherapy may be diverted into this rabbit hole while the underlying hidden problem of ADHD remains unaddressed. A rabbit hole in this context is a therapeutic effort based on a false premise that does not lead to lasting improvement.

Uninformed efforts to address the difficulties of ADHD are akin to attempts of Sisyphus to roll the stone up a hill. For those not familiar with Greek mythology, Sisyphus was a king punished by Gods for not being truthful. He was compelled to roll a large boulder up the hill, only to see it roll back again. His punishment was to see his labors being nullified and having to push the boulder up again to his great consternation and frustration.

Another analogy is to compare the ADHD condition to darkness in a room. The person does not realize that there is a light bulb that is not working and tries to do everything but replace the light bulb. The fused light bulb is the lowered neurotransmission in the prefrontal lobes. The enhancing of catecholamine neurotransmission in the prefrontal lobes by medications is analogous to fixing this circuit problem of the dysfunctional bulb. This analogy seems appropriate given our current understanding of the causes of ADHD.

As mentioned earlier, the making of a diagnosis often comes as a great relief to the individual. They are able to put some context to their problems and regain some hope again. They are surprised by the efficacy of the treatments and the effortlessness of sustaining drive and focus that was so elusive before. There may initially even be some level of euphoria when the condition is recognized and treatment is begun

The high expectations do need to be tempered by the fact that some habits tend to remain and there may be some tendency to slip into older disorganized ways of doing things. They should be encouraged to utilize their best efforts and not be intimidated by their new found success or minor setbacks.

On some days, just as with everyone else, there may be pressing emotional issues that distract them. This is normal and not every day is the same. Ultimately however, their overall level of functioning will improve.

ARE THERE ARE ANY TESTS FOR ADHD?

There are no specific blood tests or other biological measures for ADHD. Various attempts have been made to create tests of vigilance such as the TOVA and quantification of EEG patterns. These however have not been always reliable and conclusive when it comes to diagnosing ADHD. The individual may can summon their wits and perform in an adequate enough manner on tests of vigilance for short periods of time. They may still however have significant impairment at other times in their day to day life.

The best diagnostic tool is often a good history obtained from the individual and teachers, parents or other family members. This combined with the clinical interview and observation may provide a more sound basis for a diagnosis. The self-rating scales and observer rating scales are also very useful. The most common rating scale is the Conner's rating scale. This and the other scales are mentioned later. Some online ADHD rating scales are also available. One can search for them by key words "Online ADHD rating scale".

WHAT IS TOVA?

TOVA is an acronym for "test of variable attention". The patient is challenged to make time bound responses to various directions given on a computer screen. It is based on the premise that ADHD individuals will have a harder time concentrating and following directions and the individuals without ADHD will do better. There is some data from persons with ADHD and without ADHD to substantiate this claim. It is utilized sometimes by clinicians to get "objective" data about attention deficit. Other clinicians rely on and prefer observation and collateral history in making their diagnosis. It appears that some individuals can do well on the test but may still have significant impairment due to ADHD.

CAN NEUROIMAGING BE USED FOR DIAGNOSING ADHD?

Although, there are neuroimaging correlates of ADHD, PET scans are not a viable way to diagnose this condition. ADHD is more than a picture on a screen. The entire biopsychosocial context needs to be reviewed including any dysfunction when considering the diagnosis of ADHD.

So, the common diagnostic approach is to rely on the clinical interview. It is still the best approach. It takes into account the reported symptoms by the patient and the associated dysfunction. In children, the hyperactivity is usually visible during the interview. In adults however, the clues may not be so obvious during the interview. The information obtained from collateral sources such as teachers, spouses or parents is factored in. The overall level of dysfunction in more than one area of the life of the individuals is given significant weight in establishing the diagnosis.

ARE PERSONS WITH ADHD LESS LIKELY TO PURSUE AND COMPLETE HIGHER STUDIES?

Yes, this statement is sadly true. Individuals with ADHD are less likely to pursue and complete higher studies. A review of the literature suggests that anywhere from 2 to 8% of college students report symptoms of ADHD. Even some bright students, who may have managed to cope with ADHD earlier, often find themselves overwhelmed by the academic demands of the later college years.

College students with ADHD tend to have on average a lower grade point average, and a higher risk for being on academic probation. They tend to have difficulties in taking timed tests.

They also have difficulty finishing projects and assignments on time. They have also been found to have a higher rate of cigarette smoking and impairment due to alcohol or illicit drug use.

This risk for these risk behaviors is lowered when treatment is provided for ADHD.

IS THERE A RISK FOR OBESITY IN ADHD?

There is evidence that there may be a correlation between obesity and ADHD. Both of these conditions have an element of psychic and emotional impulsivity. The literature suggests a complex relationship between ADHD and obesity. There are changes in the dopamine receptor distributions in the prefrontal cortex and the hypothalamus that correlate with ADHD. The hypothalamus acts as a thermostat for regulating many functions such as hunger, satiety, thirst and various endocrine secretions. The cited changes of ADHD in dopamine receptor distribution may affect the regulatory setting for satiety and appetite that in turn may increase the risk for overeating and obesity.

CAN STIMULANT MEDICATIONS BE USED IN A PERSON WITH ADHD AND HYPERTENSION?

If the person's blood pressure is controlled on current medications, it is relatively safe to utilize stimulant medications for ADHD. It would be prudent to obtain vitals at each follow-up visit while the treatment of ADHD is being adjusted.

WHAT IS THE SCIENCE BEHIND THE DIAGNOSIS OF ADHD?

In individuals with ADHD, a few brain structures such as the prefrontal lobes, the caudate nucleus and the globus pallidus have been noted to be smaller in size when compared to the brains of individuals without ADHD.

Minor EEG changes may be noted in some children. ADHD children have a preponderance of slow theta waves in the frontal lobe EEG tracings. With ADHD medications, the brain wave patterns are noted to change to more normal patterns.

Some subtle neurological signs are noted at a greater frequency in individuals with ADHD. These are also called soft neurological signs. Examples include problems with motor coordination, difficulty in age-appropriate figures drawing, problems with alternating hand movements and right left discrimination problems. Ambidexterity is the ability to use both the right and left side of body for activities such as writing or throwing. Ambidexterity may also be present in greater preponderance in children with ADHD.

ADHD is a heritable condition. The presence of ADHD symptoms in close family members can be a clue to its presence in a person.

ADHD is more common with certain genetic mutations and anomalies. During the physical examination, one must be vigilant for any atypical or unusual facial features such as mongoloid slant of the eyes, smaller cranium, large ears or other abnormalities.

Syndrome such as fetal alcohol syndrome and Fragile X syndrome are associated with higher rates of ADHD and have a distinct appearance. A phenotype is the visible manifestation in the body and facial appearance of an individual. Genotype is the unique genetic pattern of an individual. Certain genotypes (unique genetic patterns) are associated with distinct phenotypes (facial and body appearance). Fragile X syndrome for example may be suspected with a phenotype of large ears and Trisomy 21 (Down's syndrome) is associated with an upward slanting eyes and other distinctive features.

ADHD AND CHILD ABUSE
RISK

The child with ADHD can be difficult to direct and teach. This may lead to frustration and anger on part of the parents and caretaker. This anger at the child is often generated by the perception that the child's behaviors are totally willful. Through education, the parent can better understand the difficulties and take a more compassionate approach to molding the child's behavior. With appropriate interventions and treatment, the behavior of the child can improve. This lessens the risk for abuse in the future.

Parents, teachers and caretakers need to keep in mind that ADHD is a biological condition strongly influenced by genetic and environmental factors. ADHD is not the result of deficient parenting although that certainly does not help. ADHD is also not related to the "badness" of a child. Effective treatments with medications and other therapies and interventions can bring improvement in the difficult behaviors caused by ADHD. And although bad parenting does not cause ADHD; it can exacerbate or worsen the symptoms of ADHD.

This happens if parents of ADHD children become frustrated and become more coercive, overly critical, and rejecting of the child's behaviors, which the child perceives as a rejection of them.

Education and awareness allow for acceptance of the child and their difficulties with a more tolerant attitude. Training parents about principles of behavioral therapy gives them a tool that is useful in managing difficult behaviors.

The removal of distractions from the environment is also helpful. A consistent application of behavioral therapy principles along with unconditional positive regard of the child can make for lasting improvements.

It is better for both the mother and father to come to an agreement about any behavioral plan so that there is no conflict. Such agreement can provide the consistency that is needed for the plan to work.

Dealing with the complications caused by behaviors of the child at school and at home can place an added burden on all family members. There may be stress due to the extra time needed for dealing with the ADHD child. This can lead to less time with other children and less time for the parents themselves.

It is vital at such times to not get angry or blame the child for the difficulties caused by ADHD. It is ok to talk about the stress to each other but no discontent should be shown to the child. The key may be to schedule time for the other child or children and for each other. The focus should remain on getting adequate help for the individual, encouraging compliance and complimenting every gain that is made.

It is helpful to take the children to the park or a similar setting. In such an environment, the child or children can run about while allowing the parents time with each other while they keep a watch. Hyperactivity is allowed an appropriate outlet through running and play in such settings.

Useful Skills to Teach Children with ADHD

Teach your children to prepare for the next day

Teach them to do one chore at a time

Teach to break a big project into smaller subtasks

Offer encouragement and support to reinforce skills

WHY ARE ADHD PROBLEMS MORE NOTICEABLE AT BEGINNING OF THE SCHOOL YEAR?

ADHD problems can worsen at the beginning of the school year. This may be related to the following:

1. Anxiety about the ability to form new friendships

2. Anxiety about being able to perform to expected standards

3. Worry about acceptability and possible critique of the child by teachers and others.

Anxiety about all these issues at the beginning of the school year can make the problems of sustaining attention that much more difficult for the child with ADHD.

How can ADHD lead to anxiety, depression and avoidance of school in children?

Most children with ADHD experience some difficulty at school.

Children with the hyperactive, impulsive type of ADHD can be intrusive and disruptive and be at risk of having disciplinary actions taken against them. This can sometimes lead to expulsion from the class or the school in the more extreme cases. On the other end of the spectrum are children with symptoms of inattention and daydreaming.

Children may grow anxious or depressed due to their dysfunction in school. This may be exacerbated by a harsh word from a parent or a routine reprimand from a teacher.

The child may subsequently become anxious about return to school. They may feel shamed by their disability in some cases. This anxiety can be expressed at times through physical symptoms. Another name for this phenomenon is somatization. The physical symptoms produced due to emotional stress are called psychosomatic symptoms. Such symptoms serve the purpose of generating an excuse to not go to school. The child may not be aware that these symptoms are caused by their emotional distress.

When asked, the child may not be totally aware of their anxiety. When a sensitive inquiry is made however about their ability to stay on task in class, more useful information may be forthcoming. The treatment for such school refusal is to treat the underlying disorder of ADHD. A separate session with the teacher and parents to provide information about ADHD is useful.

The role of structure in the environment and the removal of distractions is emphasized.

Most teachers in western nations are well educated about ADHD and often recognize it before anyone else.

Many teachers in other countries see it as a discipline problem. The inability to comply with instructions is misinterpreted by some to be a sign of insubordination to authority. Physical punishment is sanctioned in some countries. The teacher in the cloud of ignorance may resort to physical punishment to "correct" the child.

In addition to the emotional trauma of physical abuse, such physical punishment may exacerbate the symptoms of ADHD.

It is the cruelest form of child abuse wherein the child instead of receiving help is punished for having an illness over which they have little control.

An educated teacher on the other hand can be the one that initiates the referral for an evaluation. Treatment with medications and counseling can turn the situation around for the better.

WHAT ARE THE CAUSES OF ADHD?

Our understanding of the causes of ADHD is incomplete and still in a state of evolution. It has not been localized to any one factor or to any one gene. Having said this, it is possible to identify many risk factors that have been associated with a higher likelihood of ADHD.

Diagram: Factors Associated with ADHD

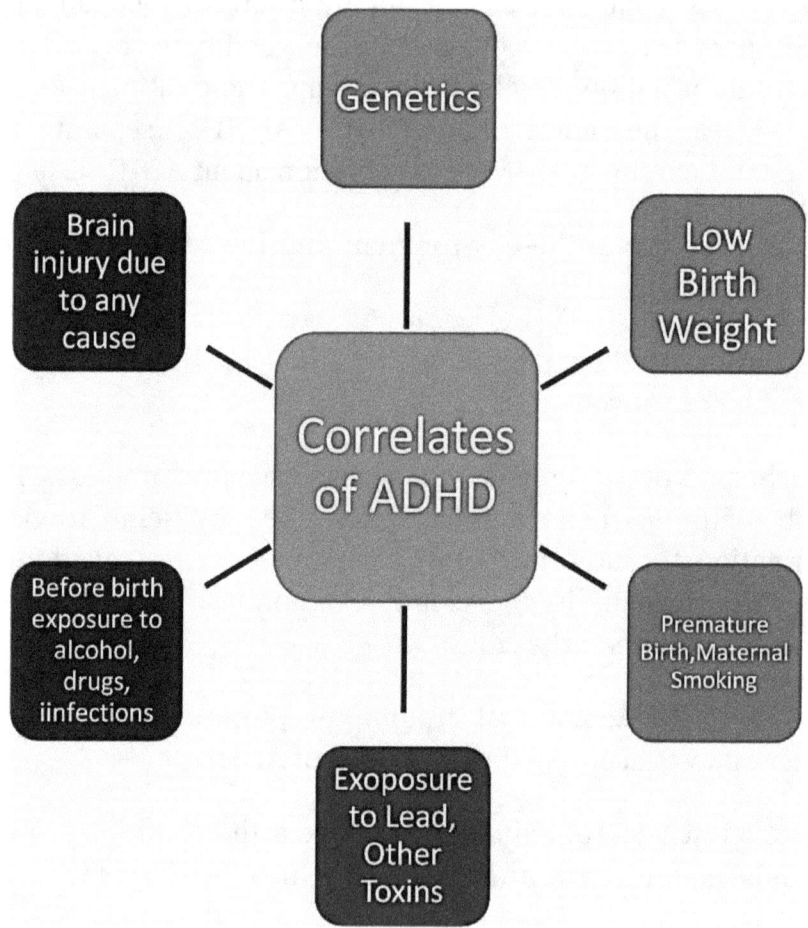

The genetic risk of ADHD is most likely polygenetic. This means that the risk may stem from more than one gene. These genes most likely are distributed on different chromosomes. Genes are small molecules that are embedded on chromosome and are carriers of genetic information that is passed on from generation to generation.

Chromosomes are long thread-like structures found in the nucleus of every living human cell and have sequences of different molecules embedded in their structure. These include genes but also other material whose function is said to be "silent."

A subtle variation in the genetic make-up of an individual can confers a risk for disease or for health. The science of genetics is fascinating and contains much that still unknown. We do know that ADHD is one of the diseases that is genetically transmitted. The diagnosis is shared more frequently by twins. This is called concordance. Concordance is higher in family members that are genetically closer indicating a genetic correlation with the condition of ADHD.

RISK FACTORS FOR ADHD

Smoking during pregnancy by the mother

Use of alcohol by mother during pregnancy.

Premature birth

Low birth weight

Exposure to lead

Low serum zinc levels

Low serum iron levels

Malnutrition due to any cause

Neglect and abuse during childhood

NEED FOR DILIGENCE WITH DIAGNOSIS

The diagnosis of ADHD should be made with due diligence and not in haste. It should only be diagnosed if the criteria for the condition are suggested by the life history and clinical presentation of the person being evaluated.

The criteria require that there should be dysfunction due to six or more symptoms related to ADHD in two or more settings. Another criteria is that this dysfunction should have lasted for six months or more.

MEDICAL WORKUP FOR ADHD

A medical review and workup is indicated for the following three reasons:

1. To rule out vision or hearing problems

2. To rule out medical or other psychiatric causes of attention problems

3. To establish that there are no contraindications to treatment with medications.

Some ADHD medications may interact with cardiac conduction, or affect the seizure threshold. The ADHD medications may also interact with other medications that the patient is on.

There are differing opinions on what kind of laboratory workup should be ordered for the patient suspected to have ADHD.

If clinical evidence indicates a medical condition, specific tests may be ordered to assess the severity of that condition. If there are abnormal physical or facial features, chromosomal karyotyping (analysis) may be ordered to rule out chromosomal diseases such as fragile X, Down's syndrome or others.

If a patient is found to have a chromosomal disorder, they may sometimes have cardiac or other anomalies. These should be screened for as well.

Some centers have a standard workup protocol that includes the following:

CBC (Complete Blood Count), CMP (Comprehensive Metabolic Panel), TSH (Thyroid Stimulating Hormone), Urinalysis and an EKG. Other specific tests such as pregnancy tests or tests for metabolic disorder, may be ordered as indicated.

Sometimes, tests to rule out the presence of roundworms may be considered if clinical evidence suggests a risk for these conditions. If malnutrition or malabsorption is suspected, serum levels of B12 and folate, and other micronutrient may be tested. If heavy metal toxicity is suspected, appropriate labs for this can be ordered. If there is history suggestive of a seizure disorder, an EEG and brain imaging may also be ordered by the physician.

A list should be made of any medications that the person is taking. It should be thoroughly reviewed as certain sedating medications, certain anticonvulsants and medication with anticholinergic side effects can have an effect on attention, cognition and concentration.

A collateral history can be tremendous aid in making the diagnosis of attention deficit hyperactivity disorder in children as well as adults. Consequently, the clinician should get a collateral history of functioning in the home and at school.

The parents are provided either a Conner's or a Vanderbilt rating scale. They are directed to have the teacher fill this out and to bring it back on the subsequent visit. There are versions of these same scales that the parent or guardian fills out. Hence the evaluation of ADHD may take more than visit in order to gather the collateral information.

DISCUSSING OPTIONS FOR TREATMENT

Once the diagnosis of ADHD or ADD is confirmed, the patient and the doctor should discuss the different treatment options. Both pharmacological and the non-pharmacological options should be discussed. The minor should also be included in treatment planning as they may have a sense of their need and are hopeful of getting help. Behavioral interventions should preferably be discussed with the parents alone. Cognitive behavioral therapy can be discussed with adults or the older adolescent that is capable of deeper insight. Reading materials can be helpful for the family and the patient.

If medications are chosen, a follow-up visit is scheduled in 1 to 2 weeks to assess response and any side effects.

How do children respond to treatment with medications?

Most children with ADHD do well with the right ADHD medications. The hyperactivity and impulsivity is often the first symptom to resolve followed by gradual improvement of attention and concentration. When side effects occur, an adjustment of the medication can often resolve the problem.

Is ADHD a disability?

The ADA or the Americans with Disabilities Act considers ADHD a disability. The ADA provides protection from discrimination when the person works for a businesses that employ 15 or more workers. Under this act, the employee that has ADHD may be entitled to special assistance if needed to do his or her job.

ADHD AND CO-OCCURRING DISORDERS

The incidence of learning disorders is higher in patients with ADHD. The following learning disorders may coexist with ADHD.

Developmental reading disorder

Developmental mathematics disorder

Dyslexia

Secondary disorders such as oppositional defiant disorder and conduct disorder may exist in some children with ADHD.

When adequate treatment is provided for ADHD, these behavioral problems decrease in frequency and intensity. Sometimes they totally go away.

The treatment of these behavioral difficulties requires a personalized treatment approach keeping the individual developmental history of the child in mind.

Treatment can involve allowing them to express their conflicts. This expression can be elicited in individual talk therapy or indirectly through play therapy. Any gains made in such therapy should be complimented.

ADHD AND COEXISTING ANXIETY MORE COMMON IN WOMEN

ADHD in girls is often marked by a different symptom pattern than boys. For example, it is noted that in girls, the hyperactivity component may be manifested by increased talkativeness. Also, the symptoms may be of the inattentive and distracted type. As inattention can be more subtle and more easily overlooked, the ADHD syndrome of girls tends to be underdiagnosed and thereby undertreated.

Untreated ADHD in girls has been correlated with a higher rate of depression and anxiety in later life.

If a clinician sees a woman with symptoms of anxiety or restless depression, it is useful to ask if they experienced symptoms of ADHD in childhood. They may not be familiar with the symptoms. The patient can be provided a list of the symptoms. If there report is suggestive of childhood ADHD, further data should be gathered from collateral sources. If such is present, they can be offered treatment with a nonstimulant such as guanfacine titrated up slowly. A positive response is often obtained for anxiety as well as the ADHD symptoms.

Hence, the diagnosis and treatment of residual ADHD may be the cornerstone of effective treatment in some cases of anxiety. Treatment is gratifying for both the clinician and the patient since effective pharmacological and non-pharmacological treatments are available. Treatment of the underlying ADHD not only helps with their anxiety but may help them realize their untapped potential through improved focus and concentration.

ANALOGIES FOR ADHD

ADHD is comparable to other chronic conditions such as hypertension, diabetes or asthma. They are similar in requiring commitment on part of the patient and the clinician for ongoing treatment goals. The clinician needs to provide guidance and support if there complications. He or she needs to offer encouragement and validation of positive gains and compliance.

Another popular analogy is to compare ADHD to a person with refractive error that needs eyeglasses. Sure, holding the object nearer or further away may help, but getting treatment by wearing a pair of glasses is so much easier and improves their lives in such a dramatic manner that it is illogical not to use them. The relief felt by the ADHD patient when treated is similar. Many believe that it is pointless and silly not to consider one or more of the different treatment options if they can dramatically provide relief for the symptoms and lessen the disability.

WHAT ADHD IS NOT

- It is not inattention or distractibility caused by acute or chronic sleep deprivation

- It is not inattention or distractibility caused by intoxication or withdrawal from caffeine, nicotine, alcohol, or other drugs

- It is not inattention and distractibility caused by a stressful emotional event or a stressful living situation

- It is not inattention and distractibility caused by a manic, depressive, psychotic or anxiety disorder related illness

- It is not inattention caused by pain and physical discomfort

- It is not inattention caused by medical problems such as narcolepsy, sleep apnea, partial seizures, metabolic disturbance or other medical conditions.

WHAT ARE SOME EMOTIONS THAT THE PARENT MAY EXPERIENCE WHEN THE CHILD HAS SYMPTOMS OF ADHD?

Parents sometimes blame themselves for the behavior of their children. Needless to say, this can lead to emotional difficulties for them. The parent should be assured that ADHD is a neurobiological disorder that has its roots in biology and that they have not caused it by their parenting techniques. This seems to relieve the guilt and allows for a shift of the efforts towards learning more about ADHD and of how to best help their child.

Do bright children run the risk of not being diagnosed early?

Some bright children may be able to compensate for their ADHD. They are able to learn quickly despite their short attention span. Education tasks are manageable because it requires less cognitive effort for them to master the material.

The behavior problems are tolerated or condoned because they continue to get good grades. The disorganization caused by their ADHD can be attributed to the quirk of genius or high intelligence. This may lead to the condition going unrecognized and untreated.

The individuals may run into difficulty when they go to college to pursue higher education. In higher studies, more self direction and organization is required. This may strain their ability to stay on track leading to failure or underperformance in their courses.

A detailed and unbiased exploration of childhood history along with collateral information from teachers and parents may reveal a pattern indicative of ADHD.

With treatment, these individuals can often improve their functioning not only in academic areas but in their interpersonal lives as well.

High intelligence is therefore no insurance from ADHD but may actually lead to an under diagnosis and consequent undertreatment of the disabling condition in these individuals. Some brilliant scientists have been thought to have had ADHD.

KEY POINTS ABOUT TREATMENT

It is important to keep in mind the following key points when considering treatment options for ADHD

1. Effective treatments are available

2. ADHD can be treated by a range of medications in an effective manner

3. ADHD can also be treated by cognitive behavioral therapy, and individual therapy.

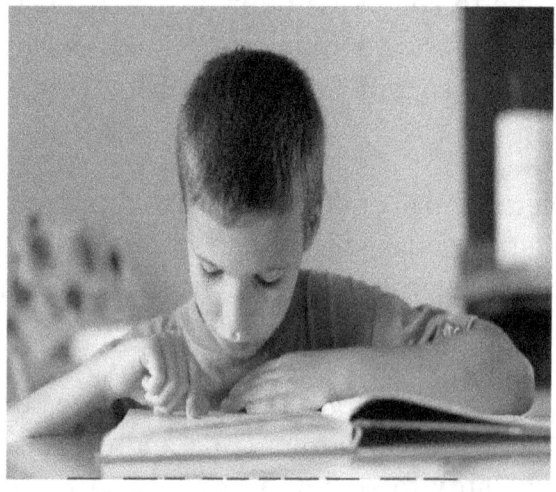

Goals of ADHD Treatment

Improve Focus
Decrease excessive motor activity
Decrease impulsivity
Reduce disruptive behaviors
Increase social adjustment

4. ADHD can be treated by bio feedback and neurofeedback

5. A combination of therapies works the best

6. Treatment compliance may be a problem due to the very nature of the illness that is marked by a lack of persistence and difficulty in staying focused and on task.

7. Family support and encouragement is very helpful in continuing treatment and keeping appointments

8. ADHD coaches can be very helpful for individualized advice and encouragement.

PSYCHOTHERAPY   IN CHILDREN

The key concepts of therapy for ADHD are:

- Education about the illness

- Teaching organizational skills

- Acceptance of difficulties

- Giving praise for desirable behaviors

- Teaching coping skills,

- Teaching to think before acting

- Making to do lists

- Teaching about limiting distractions

- The use of noise cancelling headphones may help with decreasing distractions. They are available for both children and adults.

- Use of "Thought Web" when studying- this involves taking notes and making spoke diagrams of any items related to the topic and further spokes from any of the subtopics and so on till it looks like a web. This technique helps to hold attention and also consolidate in a logical manner the different items related to a subject area.

- Help in setting up structured routines and schedules.

- Teaching parents and teachers about positive reinforcement of desirable behaviors and effective use of time outs

- Teaching kids how to wait their turn

Education and Psychotherapy: A professional counselor or therapist can help an adult with ADHD learn how to organize his or her life with tools such as a large calendar or date book, lists, reminder notes, and by assigning a special place for keys, bills, and paperwork. Large tasks can be broken down into more manageable, smaller steps so that completing each part of the task provides a sense of accomplishment.

Psychotherapy, including cognitive behavioral therapy, also can help change one's poor self-image by examining the experiences that produced it. The therapist encourages the adult with ADHD to adjust to the life changes that come with treatment, such as thinking before acting, or resisting the urge to take unnecessary risks.

WHAT IS THE FOCUS OF CURRENT RESEARCH ON ADHD?

NIMH has invested significant effort and funds to better delineate the genetics, and biology of ADHD. It has also launched various trials for objective evaluation of efficacy and safety of the standard treatments in all age groups. One of these studies goes by the acronym MTA study. This stands for "Multimodal Treatment Study of Children with ADHD".

Providing Education to Parents about What Constitutes Abuse

Some parents have misconceptions about what constitutes abuse. An abusive pattern of child rearing may run from one generation to another and be considered a normal part of raising a child. Recent media headlines of some professional athletes being abusive to their children are the clearest example of such familial illness.

It is only through education that the cycle of abuse can be prevented for the next generation.

All adults must be educated that it is not ok to strike a child for problematic behaviors. Due to the power disparity, abuse can easily get out of hand. Child abuse of any kind is a punishable offence. If the child protective services department feels that the child is danger of further harm, they may remove the child from the home to ensure safety of the child. In addition, there can be criminal penalties of jail and longer incarcerations.

If you have differences with your spouse, don't engage in any verbal or physical confrontation front of the children, as it can be deeply disturbing to them.

Educate that verbal and physical can have lasting consequences for the child. Studies indicate that abused children have higher rates of depression, self-harm and self-sabotage in later life. When the parent is educated about such dire effects, they often resolve to never be abusive again.

WHAT ARE SOME SIGNS THAT THE INITIAL DIAGNOSIS OF ADHD MAY NOT BE CORRECT?

If there is a significant mood component upon initial presentation along with disruptive and seemingly hyperactive behaviors, it is important to rule out the role of depression in causing the symptoms of seeming inattention. Children do tend to act out their depression in behavioral terms that can look similar to ADHD. Once the acute crisis and accompanying distress resolves, the secondary acting out also resolves. If the initial diagnosis of ADHD was made during an emotional crisis, it is at a higher risk for being made in error.

If mood problems are at the root of symptoms of hyperactivity or inattention, they will subside with the successful treatment of depression.

Mania and hypomania are rare in children but one to three percent of the adults may have cyclic elevations of mood. Such states are marked by hyperactivity, distractibility, and chaotic disorganization. The condition is time limited but atypical chronic presentation may be confused with ADHD. In such circumstances, a full imaging study of the brain should be done to rule out any intracranial causes such as tumors, strokes, etc. If symptoms of distractibility or impulsivity get worse, it may be a clue that the underlying condition may not be ADHD but cyclic mood disorder presenting in a manic or hypomanic phase. Treatment of the underlying mood disorder with medications such as Depakote or lithium usually helps to resolve the mood instability and also settles the symptoms of distractibility, poor concentration and impulsivity.

If there is diversion or abuse of medications prescribed for ADHD, it is a clue that the diagnosis of ADHD may have been made in error. The diversion or abuse of stimulants is infrequent in individuals with correctly diagnosed ADHD. The stimulant normalizes the catecholamine deficit related ADHD symptoms and does not produce a "high" for the individual. The use of higher than prescribed doses to get a high or rush is a sign of substance abuse and suggests that the person may not have ADHD. The use of stimulants should be withdrawn in such cases and the diagnosis should be reconsidered.

If ADHD is still suspected, nonstimulant medications such as guanfacine (Intuniv), clonidine (Kapvay), desipramine or bupropion may be better treatment options for such individuals with ADHD.

If the ADHD-diagnosed child is able to do well on some days or several days without the medications and no hyperactive or disruptive behavior are noted, one should reconsider the diagnosis.

The ADHD child may be calm and focused for short periods of time when he or she is interested in something of unique interest. If they are off medications and are able to stay focused and without hyperactivity for several days, the ADHD diagnosis should be questioned.

ADHD is not a sporadic or intermittent disorder. ADHD has a persistent and enduring presentation in the day-to-day life of the person. It presents itself in multiple settings in an unremitting manner. Any sustained resolution of symptoms should raise suspicions that the previous diagnosis may have been in error or that the condition has resolved with further development of the growing brain.

Usually, the symptoms are present in childhood and easily noticed in the earliest years of kindergarten and the early elementary school. If collateral history can not substantiate such a history, the ADHD diagnosis should be made with a great deal of caution.

In girls as mentioned, it may go undiagnosed and adult women are therefore likely to have a harder time offering proofs of ADHD in childhood. The recognition of adult ADHD or ADD in women therefore can pose a greater challenge to clinicians.

The presence of significant conduct disorder may indicate a need to rule out psychosocial stressors or abuse. Such stressors in childhood can lead to secondary acting out behaviors by the child. They are in fact the physical manifestations of the inner emotional turmoil of the child and not necessarily related to ADHD.

Another clue that the diagnosis of ADHD is in error may be the lack of a response to treatment or worsening with the standard ADHD medications.

Behavior problems caused by impulsivity of ADHD generally shows a dramatic improvement with treatment.

After treatment is initiated, it is wise for the clinician to obtain a follow-up report from teachers, parents or the spouse. They are able to recognize improvement that may not be apparent sometimes to the individual that has ADHD.

Most patients however do sense the improvement. When asked, even young children voluntarily report that the medication helps them to do better in class and at home. They may even ask that the medication be continued, as they are impressed with the benefits.

CONCERNS   OF
PARENTS

Some parents may be concerned that ADHD is being overdiagnosed and medications are being prescribed too quickly for the "problem" child, without looking deeper into the social context that the child is struggling with. The thinking is that social and environmental factors may play a significant role and the first interventions should be aimed there instead of reflexively prescribing a pill for a complex problem that is too conveniently explained by biology gone awry. There may be some merit in this argument and clinicians should take a careful social and developmental history and obtain collateral data before rushing to prescribe medications.

These concerns although valid sometimes can cause a significant delay in getting help for the children that need it for a healthy and normal development. There is a delay of almost 2 years from the time that problems are recognized and before the child is usually brought for treatment

What are things that families can do to cope with frustrations caused by ADHD?

Anger and frustration can breed amidst the dysfunction caused by ADHD.

It is important to take the steps that are needed to get help for the family member with ADHD and let go of past resentments.

The parents should remember that the behaviors are not the result of the child being a "bad seed" or malicious. Negative labeling should be avoided.

Learn the principles of behavior therapy such as praising desirable behaviors and of using rewards for goals achieved.

In addition to praise when the child is doing well, give them tangible rewards. Make every effort to catch them doing something right and applaud it! This will increase the chance of that behavior recurring.

Learn to use time out in a nonpunitive manner to allow the child to gain control

Do fun activities together with the child.

Outdoor physical activity has been shown to be helpful with ADHD symptoms.

Keep a regular predictable schedule to provide structure. Post it somewhere like the refrigerator or a bulletin board.

Let the child know of changes to the schedule in advance.

Have a preset place for everything.

Help the child learn how to use organizers of different kinds.

Give clear directions in simple language.

WORKING WITH YOUR CHILD'S SCHOOL

Let the teacher know the child has ADHD and what treatment is being provided. By making them an ally, you can help your child do better in class. Ask for periodic feedback from the teacher and share this with the doctor. This will help him or her know if a change or adjustment of medication is indicated.

If the child continues to have problems with learning, speak to a school official about having the child tested for any learning disorder. Some school districts provide for such testing.

Ask about having an IEP (Individualized Education Plan) developed for your child. Children with ADHD may be entitled to this or a similar accommodation in developed countries.

For the child struggling with certain math problems, innovative new options are available such as online lessons. Many lessons are provided for free on sites such as You Tube. The parent should verify that the sites are valid resources. The teachers may also be knowledgeable about resources for learning on the internet.

In some ways, online video lessons are perfect for the individual whose attention wavers. They can pause and rewind and replay a lesson in order to better understand the concepts that they may have missed the first time.

IF MY CHILD IS DIAGNOSED WITH ADHD, WHAT ARE THE CHANCES THAT OTHER FAMILY MEMBERS MIGHT HAVE THIS CONDITION ALSO?

The risk of ADHD being present in one of the parents is said to be about 30 to 50%. If the ADHD is marked by significant hyperactivity, conduct problems or oppositional behaviors, there seems to be some evidence that the risk for heritability may be higher.

The risk in other brothers and sisters is about 15 to 30%.

Sometimes the parent also has ADHD and needs to be treated for the dysfunction ADHD may be causing in their lives.

Treatment may improve their ability to be more helpful to their child. They are able to better understand the treatment involved and better able to keep appointments.

They are also able to learn the behavioral interventions and are more consistent in implementing them when adult ADHD does not cloud the picture.

WHAT PERCENTAGE OF ADHD GETS TREATED?

There are no exact numbers but most individuals with ADHD are not diagnosed with it and do not receive any treatment.

The diagnosis and treatment of ADHD may be understood as a tapering pyramid. The base of the pyramid represents the true prevalence, the second tier represents the ones that are diagnosed, and the third tier of the apex represents the minority that receive any kind of help or treatment. It is believed that about a tenth of adults with ADHD are recognized to have the condition (ADHD). It is only a small minority of this number subsequently pursue treatment.

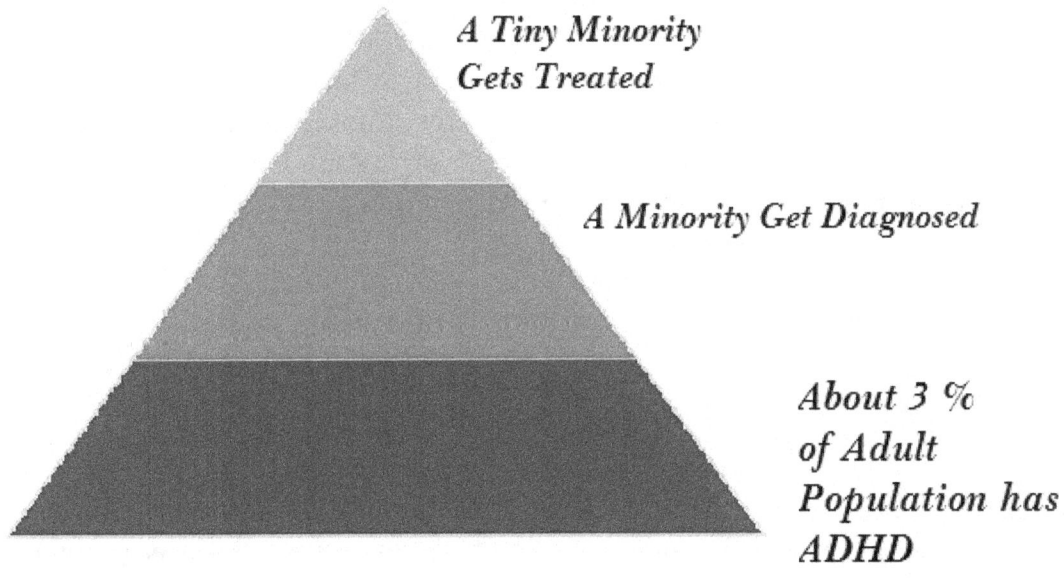

HOW CAN MY KID HAVE ADHD WHEN THEY CAN PLAY VIDEO GAMES FOR HOURS?

To understand this seeming paradox, it is helpful to understand that in the playing of videogames, there is a frequent change of focus. The video games are not challenging the ability for sustained focus. The continuing shift of focus may even make it appear that the child is hyper-focused on the activity.

ADHD on the other hand is a condition marked by difficulties with sustained attention and focus. It becomes evident in tasks where there is not a shift of focus on a frequent basis.

Such sustained attention is required in activities such as doing homework or listening to a lesson that the teacher is teaching.

SOME OTHER THOUGHTS ON TEACHING

It is helpful for the teacher to make the subject interesting and lively as possible. The teacher may improve attention by summarizing and repeating themselves at the key points in their lectures. Another strategy is of asking a question and then providing an answer. The question answer format helps in organizing focusing on the topic under discussion.

It helps if the teacher provides breaks every 15 minutes. This can be done for 2 to 3 minutes by providing a humorous or interesting anecdote to illustrate a point.

It allows the ADHD brain to "recharge" for the next leg of the lesson.

Great teachers may utilize such teaching tactics at a conscious or unconscious level. A great teacher can make even an opaque or dense subject translucent and lucid for all. They bring knowledge not only to the individual with ADHD but everyone that is trying to learn about that subject or topic. A great teacher can make learning thrilling and almost effortless.

WITH SCHOOL REFUSAL, WHAT OTHER PSYCHIATRIC CONDITIONS NEED TO BE RULED OUT?

When a child adamantly refuses to go to school, there are some other conditions that need to be ruled out.

One of these is Separation Anxiety Disorder. It is linked to a great fear in the child of being away from the parent or caretaker. They may feel terrified and doomed when left at school and may cry for long periods of time.

This condition is often linked to anxiety about a parent's health or condition. It is related to the fear of somehow losing the parent or of harm coming upon the child. The sense of doom and foreboding is significant and can be very frightening for the child.

The usual way to deal with this is to have the parent be present in the class for a period of time and then gradually decrease the amount of time spent by the parent in class until the child learns to be less anxious about the absence of the parent.

In due time, the child is able to comfortably go to school and stay there without being anxious or distracted by his or her worries.

In extreme cases, a low dose of anti-anxiety medication may be helpful.

Sometimes the child may have good instincts and the one of the parents, usually the mother, may indeed be feeling overwhelmed, stressed and depressed. Providing counseling, support, and treatment for the parent may help the parent and thereby the child.

Sometimes involvement of social agencies to help "problem solve" for the overwhelmed parent can make a big difference.

These problems may be related to marriage difficulties, housing, transportation, food, or other deprivations.

Linkage with support services can be very helpful.

By treating the parent, the child is relieved of the anxiety symptoms as well.

Another cause of school refusal may be bullying . This is becoming increasingly recognized at all levels and principals and teachers have been taking proactive steps to stem this problem. This issue gained public attention after the suicide deaths of a few children due to bullying. Some of the notable rampages by children such as at Columbine are also thought to be related to the perpetrators having been bullied.

Thus bullying is a significant stressor. It may contribute to school refusal.

If the child complains of being bullied, his complaints should be taken seriously and a meeting with the school principal may be in order to have effective action taken. The child always needs an advocate to speak for them so that abuse and bullying is not condoned or continued.

WHAT KIND OF RESPONSE CAN BE EXPECTED FROM MEDICATIONS PRESCRIBED FOR ADHD?

Response to stimulant medication occurs within hours

Hyperactivity may decrease noticeably and is usually the first symptom to improve. The improvement in attention and focus is more subtle and is noticed in a more gradual manner. The improvement may be reflected by enhanced productivity at work or by a gradual improvement in school grades.

Another clue about improvement may be a greater organization in their personal and professional lives.

CONTROVERSY ABOUT TREATMENT OF ADHD

This is most likely because the causes of ADHD are not well understood and the manifestations and expressions of ADHD are complex, diverse and multifaceted.

Whenever there is not a clear-cut and discrete relationship of a single cause and subsequent illness, many theories try to fill the vacuum with their own explanations of the cause, effect and solutions to the problem.

The different theories will sometimes contest each other's validity and salience. The truth may however be much like the fable of the elephant and the blind men. A dogmatic, one faceted approach may only capture one piece of the puzzle.

It is our opinion, that if understanding is to be more complete, it requires an open-minded holistic and eclectic approach to all theories and opinions. It is only by putting them together and adjacent to each other that one can come closest to an approximation of the truth.

There may not be one single answer to the cause or one single answer to the best treatment for ADHD. The cause may predominantly be of one kind in one person and perhaps a different pattern of contributing factors may exist in another person.

Depending on the cause and behavioral manifestations, the treatment that is best may also vary from person to person and needs to be individualized for the best results. Such an understanding may arrived at by looking at all the factors and trying what works best for the individual.

SURVIVAL VALUE OF ADHD GENE DRD4

There is some interesting thought on this subject. Conventional wisdom is that evolution weeds out any traits that are not useful and only allows the survival of the fittest. From this standpoint, ADHD may have some redeeming value and was preserved because it helped in the survival of the species. More specifically the gene DRD4 gene mutation has been found to have occurred around the time that the population began to emigrate out of Africa and other cradles of ancient mankind in search of new hunting grounds and resources. The DRD4 gene linked to ADHD is thought to have survived in this migrant population because it served a useful survival purpose. Others think that this mutation may have occurred first and this in turn may have made some individuals more restless and more likely to be on the move and to migrate.

For this reason, the DRD4 gene has also been called the migration gene. ADHD has been consistently linked in different populations that carry this gene. ADHD should not be seen only as a dysfunction because it may have been very functional and advantageous in some ways. For example, adults with ADHD may have been better hunters and better gatherers as their attention was able to shift and focus from one aspect of the environment to another. This may have also made them more aware of any present dangers and hence more likely to survive. They were more likely to spot game and their impulsivity may have added to their skills as hunters when a quick response was needed. Individuals with ADHD can also have unique and creative ways of solving problems. This ability to scan, adapt and manipulate the environment was a definite advantage as well when resources were scarce during certain bottlenecks in our evolutionary past.

This benefit may be evident even in modern day as evidenced by the fabulous success enjoyed some ADHD individuals who are scientists, entrepreneurs, and entertainers. They have made a great success of their lives through their restless drive to pursue unique talents in the creative arts, by their unique business ideas and by their unique inventions. ADHD individuals and their creativity may have pushed human evolution forwards towards new paradigms.

How is treatment an egalitarian act that equalizes individuals?

By providing treatment, one helps to level the playing field so that the child or adult with ADHD has an equal chance of succeeding as others without needing to expend and lay out an enormous effort to complete a task or project. By treating the neurological condition called ADHD, and by helping them to regain concentration and focus, the treating clinician in a sense levels the playing field. In such a manner, treatment can provide them the equal and egalitarian opportunity they need to succeed.

Treatment can have positive cascading positive effects on other aspects of the person's life. With treatment, the person may have an improved ability to make friends and to build social connections. These efforts may have been hampered before by the impulsivity and inattention associated with ADHD.

REASONS FOR MISSED APPOINTMENTS IN ADHD PATIENTS

The ADHD patient may cancel their appointments and not follow through on assignments. Progress may thus occur in fits and starts. This can be in part be related to an ambivalence about the diagnosis.

A second reason sometimes is the self-defeating behaviors some patients can develop over time when exposed to repeated failures. Some patients do not receive support from family members and may internalize the social stigma of "needing medications". They try to go it alone may avoid engaging in treatment for this reason.

For optimal outcomes, it is recommended that treatment with medications and cognitive behavioral therapy be continued on a regular basis.

WHAT TYPES OF PROFESSIONALS CAN HELP WITH ADHD?

ADHD is often treated by general psychiatrists and child psychiatrists. A large number of patients are also treated by family practitioners and pediatricians. Neurologists also treat this condition sometimes. These professionals can prescribe appropriate medications for the patient's individual situation. They can also monitor for side effects.

Psychologists and other therapists can provide behavioral therapy, cognitive behavioral therapy and teach organizational skills. They also work in collaboration with physicians and can help the child or adult obtain pharmacological treatment when needed.

Chapter 3
ADHD/ADD IN ADULTS

"ADD is like going through life carrying a one man band contraption, with a broken strap." — Julia Smith-Ruetz"

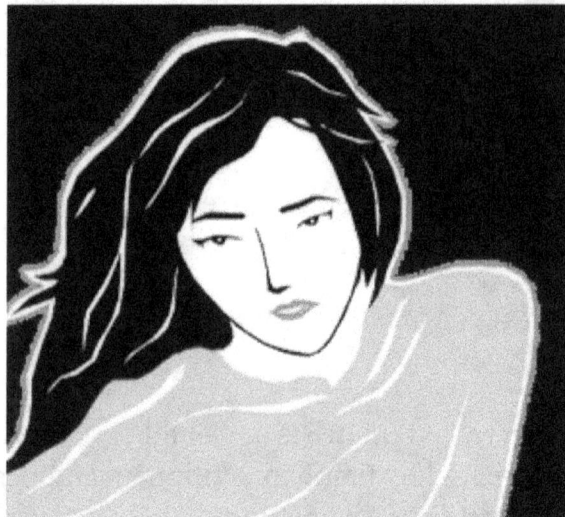

Adult ADHD Symptoms

Careless mistakes
Financial Mismanagement
Projects delayed
Assignments undone
Legal problems due to
impulsivity
Traffic fines
Poor estimate of time
requirements
Continued clutter in work and
living areas

Relationship
difficulties

Mood may be "up
and down"

What is our current understanding about ADHD and ADD in adults?

The symptoms of ADHD are a little different in adults. The hyperactivity seen in children is not as evident in adults with ADHD. The adult patient may show impulsivity in other ways. Sometimes this is manifested by reckless behaviors and impulsive decision-making.

Financial mismanagement is a common problem. They may find it hard to organize their bills or prioritize their work activities. Procrastination is common and projects may be put off until the deadline is looming on the horizon.

The *regular* frenzied last minute activity before a looming deadline can be a clue that the individual may have issues with ADHD. Their projects may suffer from a quality that is below what they are capable of.

Individuals with ADHD tend to gravitate towards jobs and occupations where a lot of planning is not needed or not possible. Examples of such jobs may be that of an EMT or a firefighter. This is not to say that all EMT's and firefighters have ADHD. Individuals with ADHD tend to be good at jobs that are of limited focus and duration. The excitement of some of these jobs can help them to organize and focus for the task at hand.

Adults with ADHD may be emotionally labile at times. This may lead to relationship difficulties. Divorce rates are higher in ADHD adults. The impulsivity and recklessness may also get them into legal trouble. The risk of incarceration is therefore higher in individuals with ADHD.

They may experience unease and anxiety from ADHD. This along with impulsivity places some of them for poor decisions in regards to the use of alcohol and drugs. Alcohol and substance abuse is more prevalent in individuals with ADHD. Treatment of ADHD with any method reduces this risk.

The impulsivity and inattention makes it more difficult for ADHD adults to sit through long meetings or carry out complicated detail oriented tasks. Adults with ADHD or ADD may also encounter economic problems that are caused by poor economic planning and poor record keeping.

Sometimes individuals with ADHD may finish other people's sentences and have difficulty taking turns in situations that require patience.

The prevalence of ADHD works out to be about 3 to 4% of the adult population in most countries.

In the United States, this works out to about 8 million adults at any given time. A significant number of them are in prisons or jails.

One of the obstacles related to diagnosing ADHD in adults is the difficulty of establishing a prior diagnosis of ADHD in childhood. This is important because a childhood diagnosis of ADHD is a requirement for diagnosis of ADHD in adults. This requirement has been relaxed to some extent because the committee for DSM V wisely agreed that an absence of a documented history in childhood does not mean an absence of a history.

ADHD can be a subtle neurological dysfunction. It is often attributed to everything else but ADHD. Often, the behaviors are chalked up to "boys being boys".

Clues about Presence of ADHD in Childhood

Clues about presence of ADHD in childhood may be indicated by a few of the following events:

a) A history of reprimand from the teacher for being disruptive in class, due to behaviors such as blurting out answers, being intrusive with other students or being resistant to reprimand and redirection.

b) Being labeled the class clown

c) A history of repeating a grade

d) Notes by the teacher that the child could achieve more if he applied himself

e) There may be a history of special interventions such as sitting in front of class.

f) History of dropping out of school for periods of time.

g) History of being in counseling for hyperactive or disruptive behaviors

h) History of treatment with ADHD medications in childhood

i) The school report cards may also have other comments about problems related to poor focus or lack of effort.

j) A history during childhood of academic failure in the presence of normal intelligence and motivation.

k) The adult may report of some current symptoms of ADHD that they can recall as having persisted from their childhood.

NOT ALL ADHD GOES AWAY BY ADULTHOOD

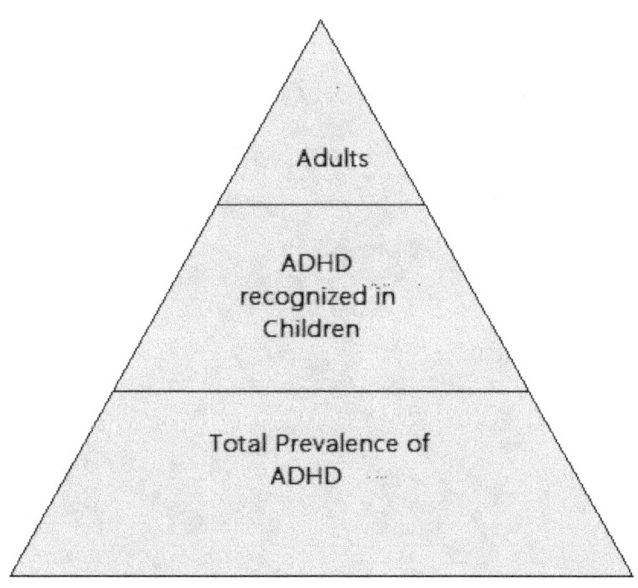

Clues in adulthood of the presence of ADHD

- A frequent change of employment

- being fired for incomplete assignments or being tardy to work.

- The adult has underperformed in their job.

- They may have had lower rank or occupational status than their talent would dictate.

- A history of having had DUIs or driving violations

- History of drug use problems

- History of smoking cigarettes

- History of difficulties in relationships and divorce

- There may be a history of ADHD symptoms in other family members.

- Impulsive decision making

- Procrastination

- Fidgetiness and restlessness

- "Zoning out"

- Difficulty sustaining attention

- Disorganization

- Misplacing things

- Losing things

- Poor management of time

- Trouble finishing projects

- Unemployment

- Underemployment

- Risk for incarceration

How is ADHD diagnosed in adults?

Adults who suspect they have ADHD should be evaluated by a licensed mental health professional. The diagnosing clinician needs to keep in mind that ADHD in adulthood may present in unique ways. The symptoms can be varied and not as clear cut and defining as the symptoms seen in children.

To be diagnosed with the condition, an adult must have ADHD symptoms that began in childhood and continued throughout adulthood. Certain rating scales can be used to elicit information.

The person should also undergo a physical exam, and pertinent labs and an EKG should be obtained. A detailed medical history and list of current prescribed and over the counter medications should be obtained.

What are some of the rating scales for ADHD?

These scales are as follows:

Child Behavior Checklist - Completed by a parent or caregiver

Conners Rating Scale for Teachers - Completed by an educator that observes classroom behaviors

Conners Rating Scale for Parents - Completed by a parent or caregiver Adult ADHD Self-Report Scale – 18 item self-report scale

ADHD Rating Scale (ADHD RS-IV)

Brown ADD Scale (BADDS)

Wender-Reimherr Adult Attention Deficit Disorder Scale (WRAADDS)

NICHQ Vanderbilt Assessment Scale - Parent informant

NICHQ Vanderbilt Assessment Scale - Teacher informant

Barkley's Current Symptoms Scale

These and other online versions are available.

ADHD rating scales should not be the sole source of data for a diagnosis!

ADHD rating scales are useful for gathering information from the teachers, parents and others. If the score on a rating scale is suggestive of ADHD, further details of the symptoms and history of dysfunction should be explored.

They need to be used in conjunction with a clinical interview and a medical examination to arrive at a diagnosis.

They should not be used as the sole method for establishing a diagnosis.

Differences between child and adult treatments

In adults, the treatment of ADHD utilizes medications as well as psychotherapy to overcome symptoms. The therapy of adults is different from therapy of children. With children, mostly behavioral therapy with rewards and consequences is used. In adults however, the therapy takes on a more cognitive and dynamic approach with the aim of understanding the thinking style. Individual therapy may also focus on anxiety, neurosis, or depression associated with past dysfunction.

Medications:

Both stimulants and nonstimulant medications are used to treat adult ADHD. The nonstimulants may pose less of a risk than the stimulants. Some antidepressant medications are also prescribed at times by some clinicians to treat adult ADHD.

Nonstimulants such as guanfacine (Intuniv) or atomoxetine (Straterra) may be the initial treatment that is offered. Stimulants such as methylphenidate or dextroamphetamines in one or the other form are also effective. Longer acting formulations of the stimulants are recommended for adults.

Examples of such long acting stimulant formulations are products such as Concerta, Adderall XR, Focalin XR or Vyvanse. It is thought the risk for abuse or drug diversion in adults is lower with the use of such longer acting formulations.

Besides these, the other nonstimulants such as clonidine(Kapvay) can be effective as well. The advantage of nonstimulants is that multiple refills can be provided and the concern about dependence, abuse or diversion is eliminated.

Antidepressants such as bupropion, desipramine and venlafaxine are also used sometimes for the treatment of adult ADHD. They are not FDA approved but are used effectively in an off label manner by some physicians. All of them have the potential to raise norepinephrine or dopamine and this property has been shown to have beneficial effects for ADHD.

Adult prescriptions for stimulants and other medications require special considerations. For example, adults when compared to children more frequently have comorbid medical problems. These problems can include conditions such as diabetes, COPD, heart disease and hypertension. They may have other medications on board to treat these conditions. The doctor treating ADHD in adults must seriously consider the interaction of the underlying disease process and any medications the patient is on.

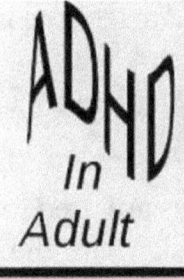

ADHD SYMPTOMS

A higher risk for the following is noted:
Having multiple projects that are delayed or never finished.
Disorganization, clutter, Late payments, fines, Traffic tickets.
Poor estimate of time.
Higher risk for impulsive act.
Criminal activity.
Misplacing things.
Forgetting things.
Missing appointments.
Relationship difficulties.
Poor planning, Financial mismanagement

STRATAGIES FOR ADHD

Have One To Do List.
Use smart Apps to Organize.
Set structure and routine in your life.
Use templates for work when possible.
Have a set place for everything such as keys, wallets etc.
Allow enough time for tasks.
Finish one project before moving to the next.
Ask another person to help stay organised.

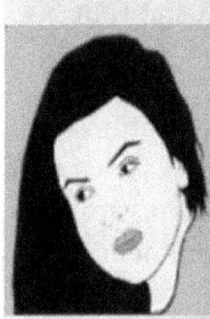

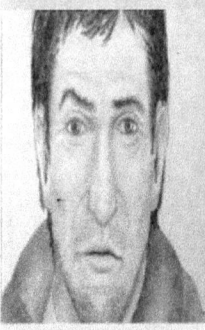

ADHD STRENGTHS

Original creative ideas.
Do well in certain occupations that require quick creative thinking.

Reasons for Reluctance in Seeking Help

ADHD is not a well-known condition for most people. Since the condition is often under recognized and unknown, it is never suspected to be a cause of their dysfunction.

The dysfunction caused by ADHD however may result in many complications. The individual may go for help and counseling to deal with anxiety or the depression. The underlying ADHD is often not recognized.

They may receive treatment indirectly for ADHD if placed inadvertently on an antidepressant that also helps with ADHD.

Some spouses recognize their husband or wife's strengths and weaknesses and will learn to help them out with their organization and goal setting needs.

There is a stigma associated with the use of stimulant medications. This stigma is prevalent towards patients and the prescribers. This is unfortunate but true and is a reason why many physicians are reluctant to treat and many patients are reluctant to receive treatment.

The national comorbidity study estimates that about 4.4 percent of the adults in the United States and probably across different countries have problems with ADHD. We have underplayed this finding and indicated a rate of 3 percent prevalence. If we take this lower conservative figure, this still represents a large number of individual that may not be aware of having this subtle but impairing neurological syndrome.

Analogy of Adult ADHD

The analogy of adult with ADHD may be similar to a person sitting in dark room due to a fused light bulb. They cannot will the bulb to function. If they try to do so, their efforts will not be very successful. What is needed is a replacement of the fused light bulb and not a lot of theorizing about the nature of darkness.

Treatment with medication helps to restore a normal balance of norepinephrine or dopamine between the synapses of the frontal lobes that is at the heart of the dysfunction caused by ADHD.

Once the analogous situation of dimmed neurotransmission in the frontal and prefrontal lobes is treated with ADHD medications, the ADHD brain finds itself coming into focus for the first time and staying on task becomes effortless. It is similar to the ease of visual perception when the fused light bulb is replaced. With treatment, the quality of their life and their performance improves as well. One success synergizes the other and they can be rescued from this vicious circle of ADHD dysfunction and emotional distress exacerbating each other in the untreated state.

A Recap

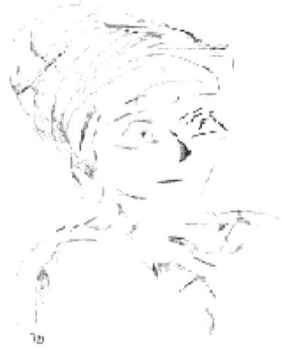

Adult ADHD Symptoms

Careless mistakes
Financial Mismanagement
Projects delayed
Assignments undone
Legal problems due to
impulsivity
Traffic fines
Poor estimate of time
requirements
Continued clutter in work and
living areas

Relationship
difficulties

**Mood may be "up
and down"**

In Men- 3 times higher
risk for arrest, fines
Procrastination
Many Unfinished
Projects
Tendency to forget
miss appointments
Misplace things often
Making impulsive
decisions without
thinking them through
Not reaching potential

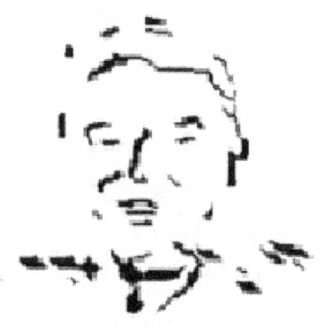

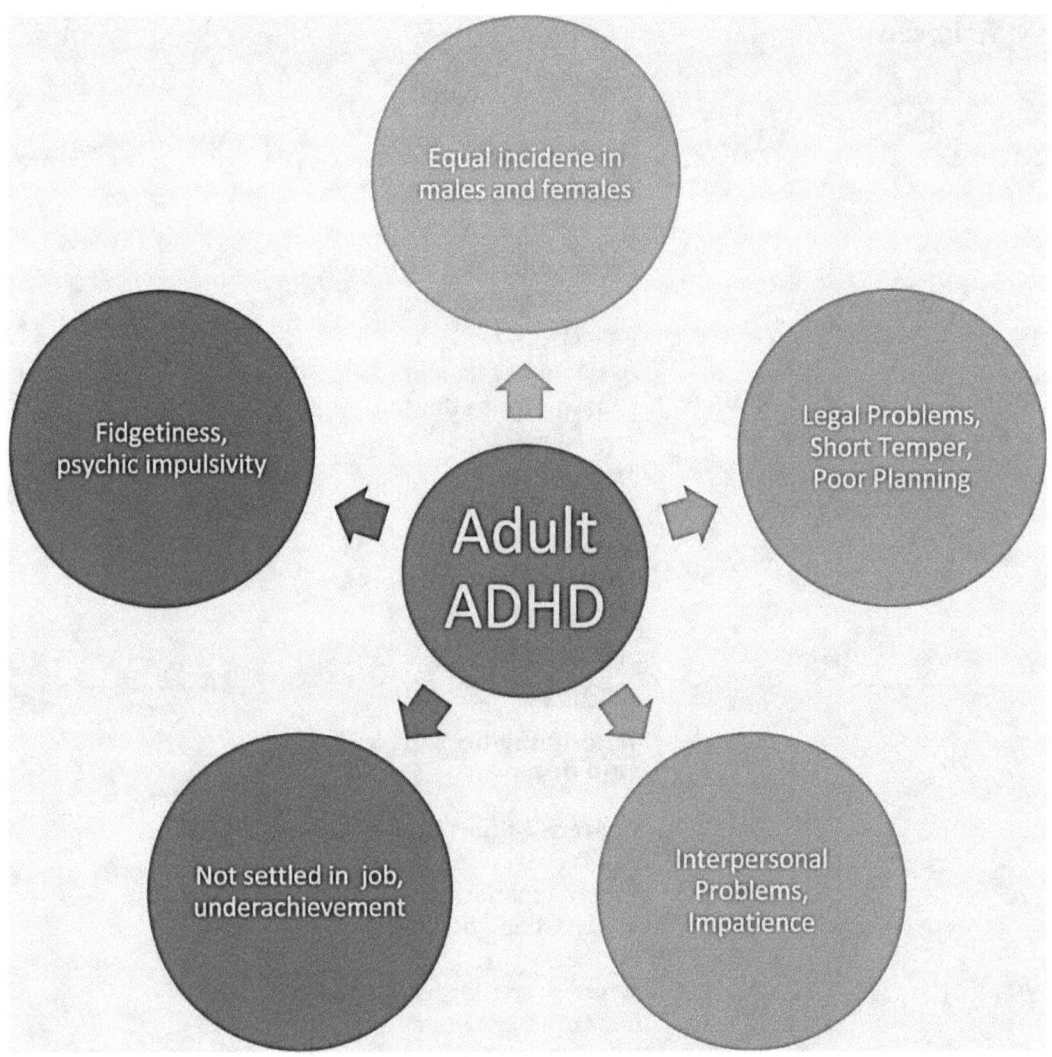

What is the Milwaukee study and what does it tell us about ADHD in adults?

The Milwaukee study is an ongoing longitudinal study following 158 children since 1977. The study is comparing the longitudinal life course of these children with the course of 81 children from a similar background but without ADHD. The study has found that just about half the children with ADHD continued to experience ADHD symptoms as adults with serious social and legal consequences for some. They were found to be three times more likely to engage in fights, destroy another person's property and be engaged in a law breaking activity when compared to the adults from the control study.

A similar study was conducted by the University of Massachusetts from 2003 to 2004 and is called the UMASS study. It compared three samples of adults from a clinic, 146 adults with ADHD, and 97 patients without ADHD. A third sample of 109 patients from the local community was also compared. It found that adults with ADHD when compared to adults without ADHD were three times more likely to engage in criminal activity. It also found that 67 percent of adults with ADHD compared to 15 percent from the other groups had trouble managing their money.

These findings underscore the fact that ADHD in adults is a treatable disorder and that it has serious consequences when not treated.

DIFFERENCES BETWEEN THE SEXES IN REGARD TO ADHD SYMPTOMS

As alluded to earlier, the traditional differences of greater prevalence of ADHD in males in childhood becomes far less skewed with age, as more females are identified and become diagnosed in adulthood.

In some adult clinical samples series, the female cases may predominate and the prevalence has been noted to be higher than the patients of the male gender. The consensus however is that the rates are the same with a ratio of 1:1.

During childhood, girls show lower rates of hyperactivity and conduct disorder than males. They more frequently have the inattentive subtype of ADHD. The quieter nature of their dysfunctions is felt to be responsible for the lower diagnosis rate by general practitioners and health care professionals. ADHD in girls is simply less well recognized and they are thus less likely to be referred for treatment.

In adulthood, the higher prevalence of anxiety and depressive disorders in women may conceal underlying ADHD. The treatment of the underlying ADHD may form the cornerstone of an effective treatment plan for resolving their anxiety and depression.

What are my options if I think I, my spouse or a family member has ADHD?

You should consult with a mental health professional that treats ADHD. There is a diverse array of clinicians that treat ADHD. They range from child psychiatrists, pediatricians, general practitioners, general psychiatrists, and neurologists. Some clinicians hesitate to prescribe stimulant medications in general because of the strict oversight by the DEA (Drug Enforcement Administration). The DEA regulates the use of all controlled substances to prevent abuse, misuse or diversion.

Most patients that are prescribed stimulants for a valid ADHD diagnosis derive great benefit. They do not become addicts and do not achieve a "high "or euphoria from the dosages of meds used to treat ADHD. Through treatment with one or the other medication and therapy, they are able to gain the competence they always had.

They for the first time, experience a sense of control and direction in their lives. Treatment can be very gratifying for both the patient and the clinician.

GOOD CAREERS FOR INDIVIDUALS WITH ADHD

Individuals with ADHD tend to enjoy tasks that require intense focus and attention for short periods of time. They also enjoy careers where their brief bursts of activity and focus are rewarded with instant gratification. This may involve the following careers.

1.   Sales, especially if outside with increased flexibility in scheduling

2.   A job or occupation in which the person has a high degree of interest

3.   EMT

4.   Firefighter

5.   Lawyer

6.   Law Enforcement

7. Emergency room workers

8. Handy Man Jobs: Individuals with ADHD tend to thrive in jobs that involve freewheeling, innovative approaches to problems solving. Some examples of this include troubleshooting jobs in the tech industry such as the geek squad, plumbing, house repairs, handyman jobs and other such vocations.

9. Independent Business: Individuals that have been taught some basics of organization and setting up of the business can thrive even if they have ADHD. They can be taught to hire people with strengths in organization and detail while they can dwell on the big picture and novel ideas for the business.

10. Some branches of the military such as Special Forces can be suitable for individuals with ADHD.

CAREER COUNSELLING AND ADHD

It is useful to provide career counseling in order to explore career options that will be best suited to the individual's aptitudes and interests, keeping in mind the ADHD limitations and strengths.

Although the above-mentioned careers work well with ADHD, any career can be successfully pursued if there is strong passion for their chosen vocation. This is especially so, if treatment for ADHD is also provided.

PROGNOSIS FOR ADULTS WITH ADHD

Adults with ADHD can learn to manage the symptoms of ADHD successfully. The success rates of such adjustments are high.

ADHD is treatable and significant relief is possible. Long-term treatment can reduce problems at home and at work, bringing patients closer to their families, and their personal and professional goals.

HOW DOES ONE KNOW IF TREATMENT WITH MEDICATIONS WILL BE HELPFUL OR IS INDICATED?

If you think you may have ADHD, don't ignore the symptoms. Even if they may not seem like a big deal to you, adult ADHD may be holding you back in ways you don't even realize. It may also be having a profound impact on the people around you, especially your family.

If you think you or someone has ADHD, it is worth the while to investigate this further and get help if indicated. ADHD is fortunately a condition that can be improved sometimes with simple interventions. A number of effective pharmacological and non-pharmacological treatments are available. If one does not want to take medications, the non-pharmacological interventions can still make a significant difference. Treatment can provide you the opportunity to be the best you can be and achieve all that you are capable of.

TREATMENT PLANNING FOR ADULTS

The patient and the doctor should be clear about the validity of the diagnosis and about the treatment goals. A plan can be developed to try a medication that is best suited to the medical condition and preferences of the patient. Psychotherapy is also recommended to recognize the thinking patterns. A measurable goal should be set such as a greater number of assignments completed, making to appointments, not being late to appointments etc.

The specific obstacles the person is facing in life can be suitable targets for treatment.

All the factors that impinge on the successful overcoming of the obstacle should be considered.

This should including inculcating a positive frame of mind, getting adequate sleep, and dividing of the bigger tasks into subtasks.

The motivating power of target dates and deadlines should be used.

Organization skills can be learned and taught.

The use of an ADHD coach should be considered.

If such a coach is not available, a family member or a friend can work as an ally to keep the person on track with their goals.

Every gain should be celebrated.

The focus should remain on success no matter how small.

Minor setbacks which are inevitable should not be dwelled on.

Follow-up with the treating doctor may be needed every one to two weeks initially and this can be stretched later to less frequent intervals. At such a time the new habits and ways of coping with ADHD will have been consolidated.

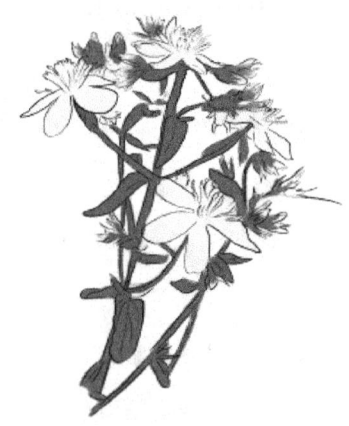

"Stand up to your obstacles and do something about them. You will find that they haven't half the strength you think they have."

Norman Vincent Peale

Chapter 4
Ruling out Other Causes of Inattention and Impulsivity

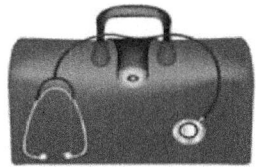

As a General Rule
Medical Conditions should be ruled
out before diagnosing any
Psychiatric Condition

Sometimes a hidden medical condition may cause symptoms of inattention and distractibility. In the adult, but also in the child, it is important to differentiate medical conditions and psychiatric conditions from ADHD. This will allow treatment to be directed towards treatment of the medical condition if it exists. The treatment of this medical condition may eliminate the problems of inattention and distractibility.

Some of these medical conditions are discussed in the following paragraphs. One key differentiating factor is often the nature of onset of the problem. Medical problems present themselves at a certain juncture in a person's life. Any attention problems related to the medical disorder are related in time to the onset of the medical problem. There is no prior history of attention problems dating back to childhood, as is the case with ADHD.

Medical and Psychiatric Causes of Inattention

- Solitary or multiple mini strokes can cause vascular dementia. They can also cause problems with inattention and distractibility. Sometimes strokes may not announce themselves with overt physical symptoms. The change in functioning is sudden however and this differentiates it from the persistent nature of ADHD symptoms from childhood.

- Unrecognized kidney disease may creep up slowly and the resultant disturbance in electrolyte balance and elevation of urea can cause problems with concentration. Inattention and frank delirium may ensue as the kidney function worsens. The long-standing history of inattention symptoms is missing.

Psychiatric Causes of Poor Attention	Medical Causes of Poor Attention
Depression- Manic syndrome Anxiety Disorders Schizophrenia Psychosis Learning Disorders Autism spectrum disorders	Petit Mal or Other seizure disorder Brain tumor Stroke Multiple Sclerosis Brain Infection such HIV encephalopathy Micronutrient deficiencies such as B12, folate, niacin, iron Metabolic disturbance causing electrolyte imablace, elevation of blood urea Elevation of ammonia Medication sideeffects from Topiramate, anticholinergic medications, others Chronic pain Sedating medications Poorly controlled diabetes Toxicity from medications Toxicity from lead, other heavy metals Developmental Delay Dementia from any cause Alcohol or other substance intoxication or withdrawl Hearing deficit Vision deficit Pinworms or lice infestation

- Epilepsy can cause lapses of attention, impulsivity and inattention during and between seizure episodes. The patient with petit mal epilepsy may be alert but distracted and have a blank inattentive look. There can be many such episodes during the day.

- If the clinical picture indicates the presence of staring spells or brief loss of muscle control, a full neurological exam, an EEG and brain imaging studies are recommended.

- Petit Mal epilepsy has a unique pattern on the EEG and encephalogram may be diagnostic.

- It is necessary rule out seizure disorder before considering treatment. This is because the use of stimulants in the presence of seizure disorder may worsen the seizure disorder or even precipitate prolonged seizures.

- These prolonged seizures are called status epilepticus and can be fatal.

- Uncontrolled diabetes can cause fluctuations of blood sugar levels, and accompanying metabolic and electrolyte disturbances. Such fluctuations may be associated with impaired attention and concentration.

- Any intracranial pathology, such as tumors, abscess or infection can cause an altered mental status with impairment of concentration.

- Infections local or systemic can cause problems with attention and concentration.

- Hormonal imbalances such as low or high thyroid hormone levels can cause attention and cognition problems.

- Unrecognized deafness of varying degree will lead to inattention, boredom and acting out behaviors.

- Unrecognized impairment of visual acuity can lead to distraction, inattention, boredom with secondary acting out behaviors.

- Subnormal intelligence and inappropriate class placement may lead to behaviors caused by frustration and an inability to understand the subject.

- High intelligence and inappropriate class placement may also lead to boredom, frustration and acting out that resembles ADHD behaviors.

- Head injury and trauma, whether solitary or repetitive has been linked to attention and cognition problems.

- Chronic medical conditions due to any cause may hamper the ability to concentrate.

- Inadequate nutrition and hunger may lead to inattention due to related anxiety and restlessness. Over the long term, micronutrient deficiencies may affect brain functioning in complex ways including issues with inattention.

- Lack of adequate sleep puts a definite damper on the ability to focus and concentrate.

- Stressors in the environment may pull attention away from a required task and towards a resolution of the stressor.

- Emotional disturbance due to interpersonal conflict makes it difficult to focus and concentrate.

- Anxiety Disorders when untreated by their very nature generate issues of distractibility and inattention.

- Depressive disorders can interfere with the ability to concentrate and to pay attention.

- In depressive states, the person may feel as if they are in a fog. They may even complain of not being able to "think".

- They may also complain of memory and concentration problems. This cognitive dysfunction associated with depression has also been called psuedodementia or false dementia.

- When the depression is treated, the cognitive fog lifts and the symptoms related to poor attention and concentrations also resolve.

- Some medications such as topirmate and those with a strong anticholinergic effect may cause issues with focusing and concentration. Anticholinergic medications often have an accompanying side effect of dry mouth. Other sideeffects such as constipation, and urinary hesitancy may also be present with anticholinergic medications.

- Any medication that elevates ammonia such as divalproic acid (Depakote) or topirmate (Topamax) may result in decreased alertness and sometimes a delirium. In these situations, there is a lack of focus and wandering attention.

- Learning disorders may present with inattention and distractibility if adequate provisions are not made to accommodate the learning deficits.

- Child abuse - These children may be frightened, apprehensive, fidgety and have difficulty sustaining attention

- Environmental Toxins: Toxic levels of certain agents such as lead have been associated with problems of inattention and poor concentration in addition to many other physical symptoms.

- Pesticides: Exposure to these in utero (while in the womb) or in later childhood has been linked to symptoms of ADHD

- Exposure to some artificial food colors and preservatives in food has been correlated with symptoms of hyperactivity and inattention.

- Pervasive Developmental Disorder - stereotypical behaviors may be seen as fidgetiness and social withdrawal may be interpreted as inattention or daydreaming.

- Tourette's Disorder–The odd sounds and motor tics of this condition may be misinterpreted as impulsivity and hyperactivity of ADHD. Sometimes ADHD does coexist and the guanfacine used for ADHD may help with some of the motor tics.

- Depression - Social withdrawal and apathy that are hallmarks of depression may be misinterpreted as inattention of ADHD. The child may at times be tearful as well and have a hard time completing tasks

- Mania - This is rare in children but present as a component of bipolar disorder in about 2 percent of adults. In mania there is indeed hyperactivity and driven quality along with increased speech and intrusiveness. This can look very similar to ADHD. A key distinguishing feature is often the lack of euphoria and grandiosity in ADHD.

- Mild cerebral palsy - Depending on the areas of the brain affected, varying levels of inattention and distractibility may be noted.

- Some obscure causes of fidgety behaviors may include pinworm or lice infestation. This may be falsely interpreted as the hyperactivity of ADHD.

ASSESSMENT AND DIFFERENTIAL DIAGNOSIS

Diagnosis	Increased Activity	Attention Problems	AH VH	Less Sleep	Mood Elevation	Unusual Fears
ADHD	Y/N	Yes	No	Y/N	No	No
Bipolar Mania	Yes	Yes	N/Y	Yes	Yes	N/Y
Schizo-phrenia	No	Y/N	Yes	Y/N	No	Yes
Depressi	No	Y/N	No	Y/N	No	No
Anxiety	May be Fidgety	Yes	No	Y/N	No	No
Epilepsy	No	Yes/No	N/Y	No	No	Y/N

- A/H = Auditory Hallucinations

- V/H = Visual Hallucinations

- Y/N = Yes/No (First choice Yes more likely)

- N/Y = No/Yes (First choice No more likely)

FURTHER DICUSSION OF PSYCHIATRIC DIFFERENTIAL DIAGNOSIS IN ADHD

Some further discussion of the following psychiatric conditions follows.

1. Psychotic Disorder

2. Bipolar Disorder

3. Depressive Disorder

4. Anxiety Disorder

5. Substance Abuse Disorder

The differential diagnosis from other psychiatric disorders can be obvious on most occasions.

There is however an overlap of symptoms between ADHD and some psychiatric conditions that can confound the acumen of even a seasoned clinician.

In children, the presence of primary psychotic disorder or manic syndrome is unusual and rare. In adults however, psychotic illness does occur in one to two percent of the population.

Differentiating ADHD from Schizophrenia and Psychotic Disorders

Psychotic syndromes such as schizophrenia have also been linked with frontal lobe dysfunction. Such frontal lobe dysfunction in the schizophrenic patient can lead them to also live disorganized and cluttered lives.

Attention and concentration in psychotic states may be less than normal due to more than one factor. First, there is some amount of frontal lobe dysfunction noted in process schizophrenia. In addition to this, attention may be impaired due to the paranoia and the distractions caused by active auditory hallucinations. In a state of paranoia, the person is often sensitive to environmental cues and can look distracted.

The symptoms of active psychosis are so dramatic and prominent that there is no mistaking them for ADHD.

The overt symptoms of hallucinations and disorganization of thought or speech will distinguish the serious psychotic illness.

If psychotic symptoms are noted in children or in an adult for the first time, a medical workup is recommended to rule out medical causes.

This usually includes a detailed drug intake history, physical examination, comprehensive metabolic profile, a complete blood count, a urinalysis and imaging of the brain.

Differentiating from Bipolar Disorder:

The differential diagnosis from a manic syndrome can be made by noting the absence of grandiose ideations or beliefs in the ADHD adult or child. The other cardinal feature of a mania such as the poorly connected flight of ideas is missing in ADHD.

ADHD in children on the hyperactive spectrum may have increased speech output and a seeming pressure to talk as manifested by blurting out answers. There may however not be the elation and flight of ideas that is found in mania. The sleep may be disturbed in ADHD but the degree of decreased sleep is significantly worse in the manic states.

The increased risk taking behaviors driven by inflated sense of self-worth and increased energy levels also have a different quality to them than the purely motor driven hyperactivity and impulsivity of the ADHD patient.

Anecdote provided by Professor Paramjeet Singh MD

An adult male patient AL was diagnosed with bipolar disorder based on symptoms of impulsivity, emotionality, and involvement in multiple projects from which the person would often get distracted. He was placed on mood stabilizers but did not show much in way of benefits. A careful second attempt at history collection revealed his pattern of behaviors to be lifelong dating back to early childhood. A diagnosis of ADHD was proposed even thought it was a remote diagnosis of exclusion. After discussion with other colleagues, the patient was given a trial of methylphenidate.

To the surprise of the treatment team, the individual attained significant benefits, becoming much calmer in his interactions with others. He was able to stay focused on his projects and finish them to the great benefit of his business interests.

This is a good real life example of how adult patients with impulsivity due to ADHD that may be misdiagnosed to have other conditions. They may be placed on anticonvulsants or antiepileptic's with suboptimal benefits. When placed on standard nominal treatments for ADHD, the beneficial response can be dramatic.

Both disorders share some similar signs and symptoms. The diagnosis of adult ADHD is easy to overlook. The absence of overt mania however should be a strong clue to lean away from the diagnosis of bipolar disorder.

To avoid misdiagnosis, it is important to take a careful history and explore the nature of the key symptoms. The subjective state of elation, pressured speech, word clanging or flight of ideas is absent in ADHD. Response to mood stabilizers is positive in true bipolar disorder. In contrast to the superb response to mood stabilizers for bipolar disorder, when ADHD patients prescribed mood stabilizers, the response is marginal to none and the patient may complain of significant sideeffects.

Differentiating from Depression

Attention and concentration can suffer during an episode of severe depression. The key differentiating feature is the marked sadness, anhedonia (lack of pleasure), constriction of affect, and disturbances of energy and sleep. Sleep disturbance may be related to middle insomnia and early morning awakening instead of the onset insomnia more typical of the ADHD patient.

Differentiating from Anxiety Disorder

In anxiety disorder, the child or adult may have been traumatized and suffer from flashbacks of the traumatic event. This may make the person look distracted and fidgety. There may be other symptoms of autonomic arousal such as sweaty palms, dry mouth, palpitations and tachycardia that are usually not a feature of the ADHD syndrome. The subjective state of the patient is also one of reported anxiety and this is usually not cited as a significant concern in ADHD patients.

In anxiety disorder, the child or adult may have been traumatized and intrusive recall of traumatic event may hamper the ability to focus and sustain attention. There may be other symptoms of increased vigilance caused by anxiety such as sweaty palms, dry mouth, palpitations and tachycardia (fast heart rate) that is usually not a feature of ADHD syndrome.

What are some other conditions that may look like ADHD?

Some of the following conditions should also be considered in the differential diagnosis of ADHD.

Child abuse - These children may be frightened, apprehensive. They can also be fidgety due to their anxiety and fright and in this context can definitely have difficulty sustaining attention

Reactive Attachment Disorder - This is a manifestation of the love-starved child and is produced often by extreme emotional deprivation and neglect. The child may look distracted and carry a forlorn expression. They may be extremely shy, withdrawn and look internally occupied. At other times, the child may try to "earn" love by an exuberant and cheerful friendly presentation accompanied by hugs or other signs of affection towards relative strangers.

This seemingly extroverted child that seeks love from any stranger may be misinterpreted being intrusive and impulsive for approaching others without inhibition or stranger anxiety.

Deafness and vision problems may cause the child to appear lost and unfocussed.

Auditory processing problems - The child may be distracted due to poor comprehension of spoken words.

Learning Disorder - The child may have difficulty keeping pace with other classmates. He or she may be fidgety or bored and appear distracted by random stimuli to relieve the boredom.

Seizure disorder: Some seizure disorders such as petit mal may be associated with staring and lapses of attention and the child may appear to be daydreaming and inattentive.

Hyperthyroidism: These children may be hyperactive, irritable and distractible as well.

Mental retardation - The child may look inattentive and distracted due to the topic being too difficult for them to understand. Placement in special education classes with less challenging material helps to decrease such inattention.

Malnourished, abused or sleep deprived children – Such situations are pregnant with many potential causes for dysfunction. Malnutrition can interfere with cognitive processing. Low levels of iron and zinc related to malnutrition have been associated with ADHD. Anxiety syndromes related to trauma and abuse can cause much disruption on many levels. Any sleep deprivation can lead to inattention and somnolence during class.

Signs of abuse may include such features as bruising, unexplained injuries, erratic pattern of absences, picking up scraps of food, withdrawn or overly friendly behavior as mentioned before.

Physical Exam Findings in ADHD

In ADHD, some soft neurological signs may be noted such as mild incoordination in movements. At other times, ambidexterity and brisk reflexes are noted. Ambidexterity is the ability to use both hands almost equally well.

A physical examination may also provide clues about any cardiac defects by the nature of the heart sounds on auscultation. This is important to rule out, as there is an elevated risk of adverse side effects in those with heart disease.

Patients with structural heart disease are at a higher risk for arrhythmias and sudden death without medications. With medications, this risk may be higher.

A baseline EKG is recommended to identify any risks. Some centers include the following labs as part of the pretreatment laboratory workup: a CBC (complete blood count), a CMP (comprehensive metabolic panel), and a urinalysis along with a test of thyroid function such as TSH. An EKG is also ordered by some to rule out any cardiac problems. This is recommended if the history or exam findings raise a cardiac concern.

An EKG is also recommended on any patient over age 40.

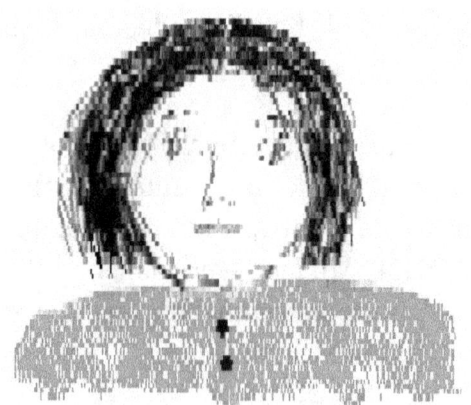

ADHD/ADD SYMPTOMS IN ADULTS

Poor Attention
Impulsivity
Restlessness
Poor Organization
Tendency to lose things
Procrastination
Trouble finishing tasks
Forgetfulness
Underperformance in Career
Underperformance in Higher Schooling
Interpersonal problems related to failure to fulfill obligations
Higher incidence of legal problems

Chapter 5
Pharmacological Treatment of ADHD

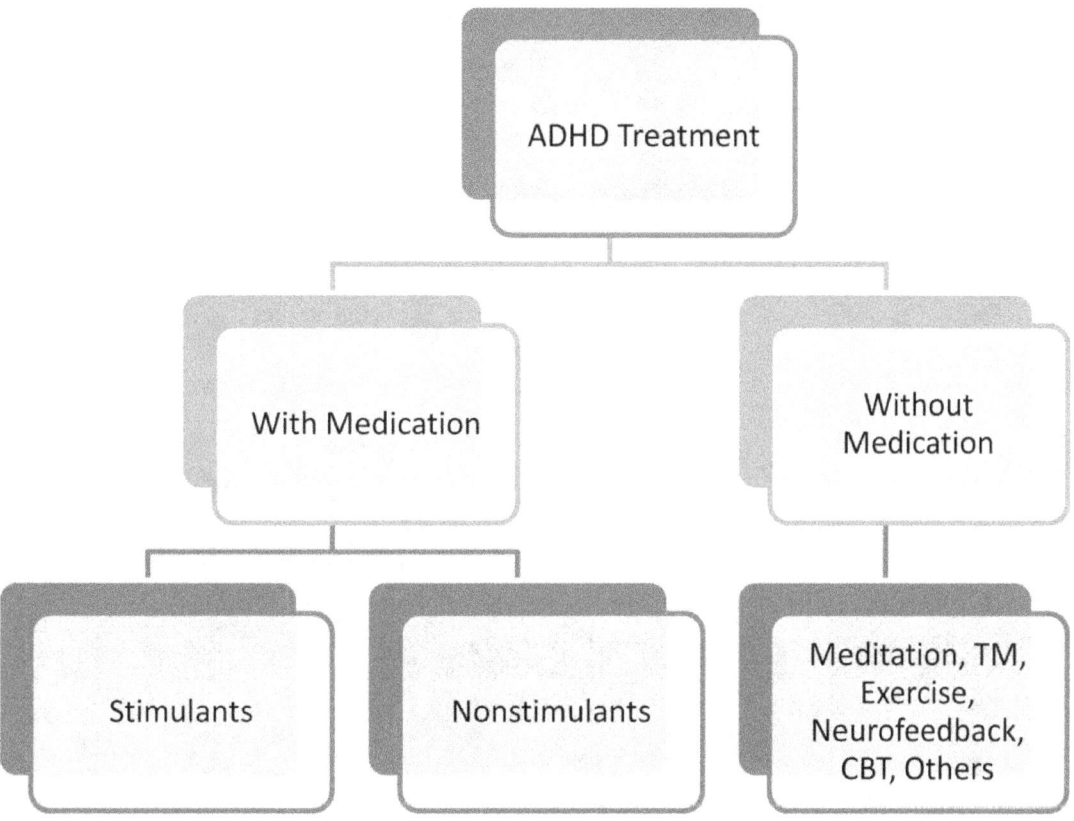

A diverse array of treatment choices is available for the treatment of ADHD. These choices are broadly classified into the medication and alternative or nonmedication categories. In general, as is the case with most other chronic conditions, a combined multimodal treatment approach is better than a single mode of treatment. For example, medications for ADHD work better when combined with a behavior program than treatment with medications alone.

Within each of the broad categories, be it medications or alternative therapies, a number of different choices are available. Each choice of treatment needs to be considered carefully as each has its pros and cons.

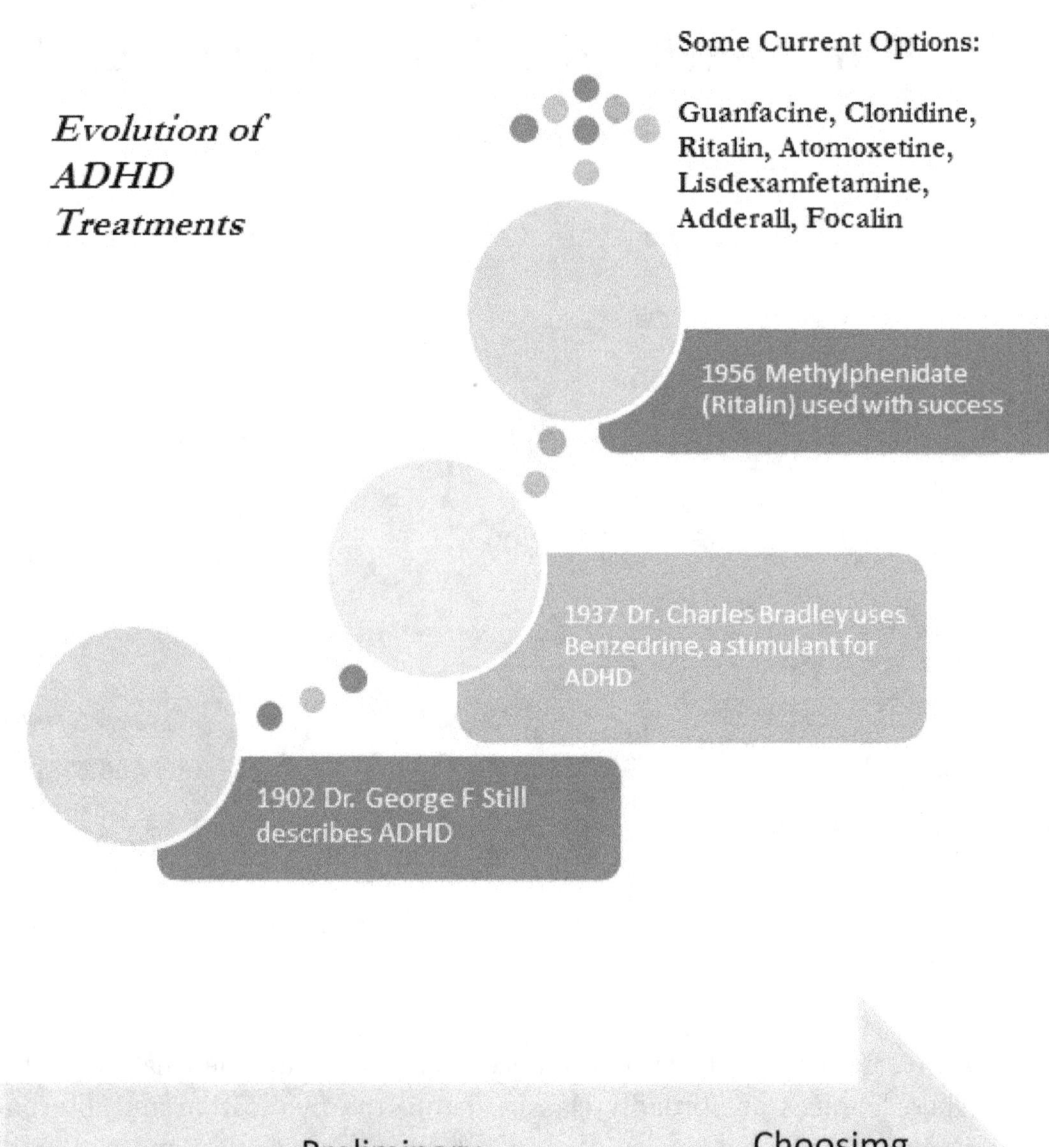

Evolution of ADHD Treatments

Some Current Options:

Guanfacine, Clonidine, Ritalin, Atomoxetine, Lisdexamfetamine, Adderall, Focalin

1956 Methylphenidate (Ritalin) used with success

1937 Dr. Charles Bradley uses Benzedrine, a stimulant for ADHD

1902 Dr. George F Still describes ADHD

Symptoms · Preliminary Workup · Diagnosis · Choosimg Treatment

Stimulant medications such as methylphenidate are the mainstay of treatment of ADHD. They have proven their efficacy in numerous trials. In recent years, the pharmacological options have broadened with the arrival of newer formulations. Some of these are older drugs packaged and formulated in new ways. Others are relatively new options. These new options include the nonstimulants guanfacine, clonidine and atomoxetine.

Even though, the stimulant medication are often used with efficacy; they may not work for every patient or may be contraindicated. The arrival of the nonstimulants therefore is a welcome addition.

Non-stimulant medications may also be preferred by patients and families when there is a risk for addiction or abuse. For such situations, these medications fulfill a useful role as effective alternative treatment for ADHD.

If one medication does not work, a different medication may be effective even if they belong to the same class. There is no one dose or one medication that will be effective for all individuals.

It is important to combine medications with other non-pharmacological interventions that are discussed in the next chapter. These are: cognitive behavioral therapy, behavioral therapy and individual therapy among others. Both sets of interventions complement each other and aid in the relief of ADHD symptoms.

The clinician should discuss the potential benefits as well as the risks of taking the nonstimulant and stimulant medications such as Adderall, Dexedrine, Vyvanse or Methylphenidate.

Stimulant medications should be avoided in individuals who have had problems with substance abuse in the past. There is a higher risk for abuse and diversion in such patients.

Stimulant medication should also be avoided in individuals who have been diagnosed with bipolar disorder, schizophrenia or schizoaffective disorder. They have the potential for exacerbating these conditions by increasing the symptoms of elevated mood, insomnia, auditory hallucinations, and paranoia.

It is standard practice to monitor weight gain and height in children when they are prescribed stimulant medications. If there is a delay in weight gain or height gain, it may be prudent to lower the dose of the stimulant and monitor the appetite related side effects.

Other strategies to deal with poor appetite are to offer more calories in the afternoon, evening and dinner in way of larger meals and high calorie snacks. The appetite suppressing effects of the stimulants wear off in the afternoon and appetite returns to normal.

Another strategy is to provide drug holidays during the seasonal holidays when school is off. In the United States this includes holidays such as Christmas break, spring break or the long summer break.

During such breaks, the stimulant medications can be withdrawn but the nonstimulants should continue if needed to control problem behaviors. The nonstimulant medications do not affect the appetite.

If nonstimulants like guanfacine or clonidine are discontinued, they should be tapered off and when restarted, they need to be tapered up to the previous therapeutic dose to avoid sideeffects. The tapering helps to avoid sideeffects.

Stimulant medications should be avoided in pregnant women and those who are lactating and nursing infants.

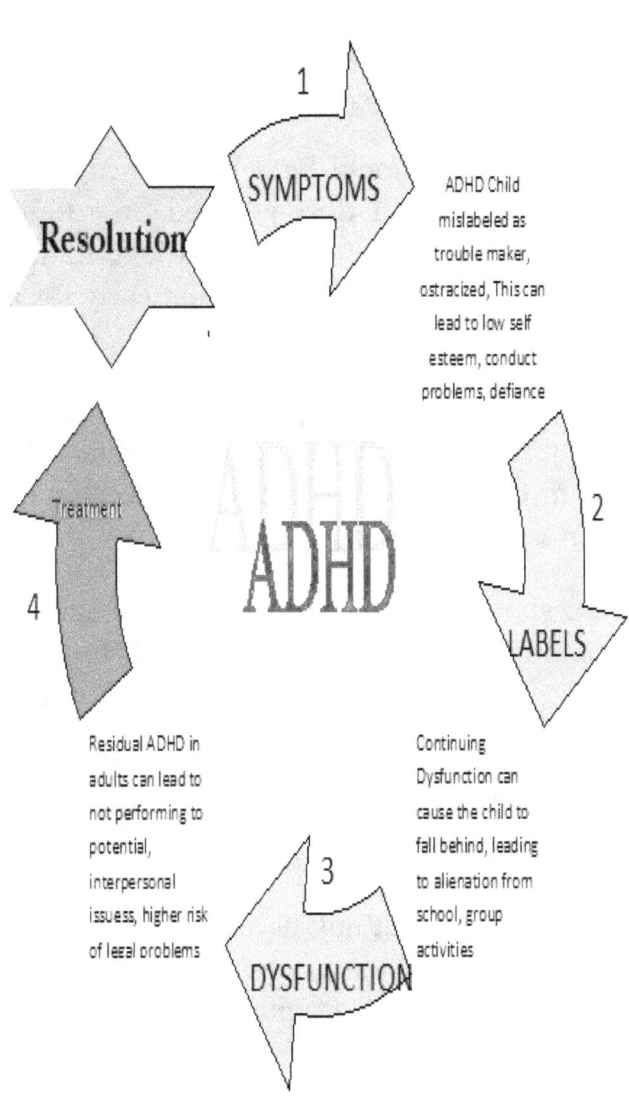

1 SYMPTOMS

ADHD Child mislabeled as trouble maker, ostracized, This can lead to low self esteem, conduct problems, defiance

Resolution

ADHD

ADHD

Treatment

4

2 LABELS

Continuing Dysfunction can cause the child to fall behind, leading to alienation from school, group activities

Residual ADHD in adults can lead to not performing to potential, interpersonal issuess, higher risk of legal problems

3 DYSFUNCTION

TREATMENT BRINGS RESOLUTION AND INTERRUPTS THE CYCLE OF DYSFUNCTION

What kind of follow-up schedule is recommended when starting the treatment of a patient with medications?

After treatment is begun, a follow-up visit should be scheduled in 1 to 2 weeks. This allows for an early adjustment of dosing based on residual symptoms and any side effects. It is useful to ask the patient to hold medication if there are any significant side effects and come in early for an evaluation.

As these patients have coped with ADHD for a significant portion of their lives, the clinician should not feel rushed in the titration schedule. The emergence of early side effects from too rapid an escalation in dosage may drive some individuals to give up on treatment.

Information from family or spouse should also be invited as the benefits of treatment may be more noticeable to family members and others before they are evident to the patient sometimes. The family is often the first to comment on the improvement in the patient.

When a stable regimen has been reached, follow-up visit interval can be lengthened to every four to eight weeks or longer.

In each session, it is important to enquire about any psychiatric or physical side effects. Psychiatric side effects may include depression and suicidal ideations in the first 2 to 4 weeks of treatment with atomoxetine.

Some clinicians insist that vitals and blood pressure be checked and monitored at every visit while others check these based on clinical discretion if the patient is otherwise doing ok.

Most clinicians prefer and favor an open-ended approach during the interview and let the patient report of their progress and of any side effects. More specific questions may be asked if there is lack of appropriate weight gain or if there are any unusual symptoms. The clinician also monitors for the psychomotor activity and any tics or abnormal movements during the interview. Any feedback from collateral sources such as teachers or parents is extremely valuable in gauging the success of the treatment.

Weighing the Benefits, Risks and Costs of Treatment

The rewards of treating ADHD are significant. The side effects of the medications can be monitored for and serious risks can be reduced by a careful medical history and examination as needed.

The treatment with generic medications can be relatively inexpensive. Some brand name formulations however can be expensive.

Serious adverse effects are relatively rare although the risk does exist for some patients with preexisting medical problems.

For a majority of the patients, the treatment costs and the risks are well worth the treatment benefits.

In recent years, more health insurance companies have begun to cover the cost of ADHD treatment. Nonformulary choices are available if the doctor can show that the formulary medications have been ineffective.

The generic brands of medications are reliable and less expensive. Even in the absence of insurance, a visit to a doctor is usually worth the benefits. Learning about the disorder and being offered nonpharmacological options can offer new avenues and resources to overcome past hurdles imposed by ADHD.

For those who cannot afford to visit a private doctor, inexpensive public health clinics are usually available for consultation about treatment.

Duration of ADHD Treatment

The duration of treatment in children varies. Some children as they mature outgrow the ADHD related symptoms. Others may require treatment through high school. Longitudinal studies indicate that about 30 to 50 percent of individuals with childhood ADHD continue to have ADD or ADHD symptoms as adults. Further validation of these studies across the globe is indicated as most of these studies have been conducted in the United States.

How long does it take to notice a response to ADHD medication?

The beneficial response to stimulant medications may occur within hours.

The hyperactivity may decrease noticeably and is usually the first symptom to improve.

The beneficial effect from guanfacine may be noted in a few days as the dose is titrated up to effective levels.

The response period to atomoxetine, venlafaxine, and bupropion may be 2 to 4 weeks but sometimes an earlier response is reported.

Psychotherapies such as behavioral therapy. Cognitive behavioral Therapy (CBT) and others have a synergistic benefit. At the risk of some repetition, creating a quiet work space and removing distractions is useful as well.

The symptoms of attention deficit are more subtle and improvement is better judged over a longer period of time by noticing an improved ability to finish tasks and an improvement in the quality of work rendered.

Another way to measure benefit is through an improvement in school grades. Teachers and family members may also notice that the person is less forgetful and more organized. Getting a collateral report from them is a good way to gauge progress.

The benefits are evident in school, work and in their personal life.

The treated person may also show a change in their personality from being impulsive and driven to being more patient and thoughtful in their responses and actions. Such changes are noted and perceived by observant family members even when not evident to the person under treatment.

A Synapse

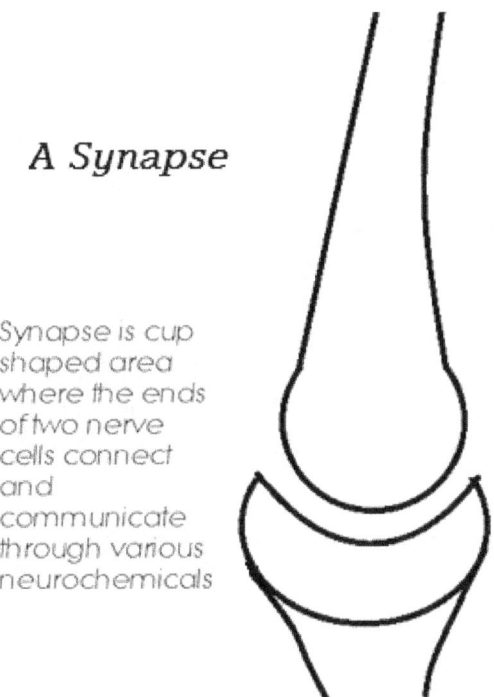

Synapse is cup shaped area where the ends of two nerve cells connect and communicate through various neurochemicals

Workup Prior to Treatment

It is helpful to get a complete history and physical and an EKG prior to starting treatment with medications for ADHD.

When the clinician is making an enquiry of past medical and family history, the following are some items to keep in mind.

Rule out any history of sudden death in family members at a young age.

Rule out any cardiac problems.

Ask about any history of allergies or adverse reactions to any medication in the past.

The use of medications called MAOI's within the last 6 weeks should be ruled out

Ask for any history of tic or Tourette's disorder that may be made worse by stimulant medications.

Labs ordered

CBC (Complete Blood Count), CMP (Comprehensive Medical Panel), UA (Urinalysis),

B12, folate levels if malnutrition is noted.

Further investigative studies may be ordered if suggested by the physical exam. These may include labs such as lead levels, chromosomal karyotyping or other tests as indicated.

CLASSIFICATION OF ADHD MEDICATIONS

The following diagram illustrates the different medication groups that are currently available.

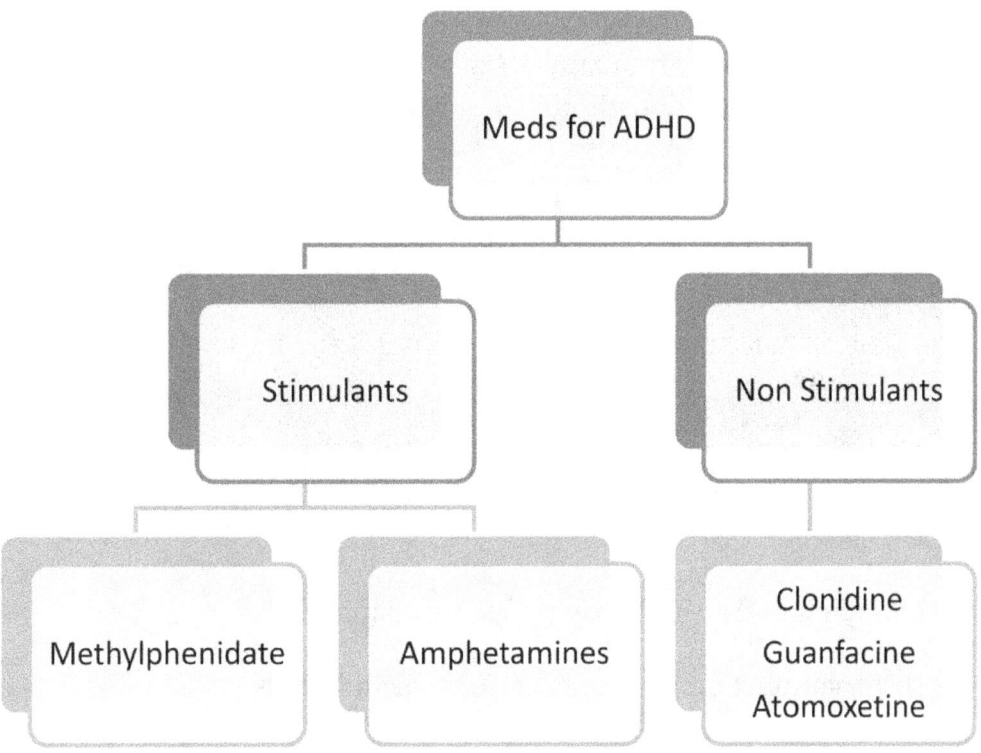

The role of medications in treating ADHD has evolved over the last 50 years. Initially, only Benzedrine was used for ADHD symptoms. This was followed by the manufacture of methylphenidate in 1956 and soon this came to be most commonly used medication for ADHD with few other choices. It is still the most commonly used medication.

Pemoline was later developed and went by the brand name Cylert. It was also used with success but had rare but serious side effect of causing hepatitis. It has currently been taken off the market in the United States. It was available generically and cheap.

Stimulants have been the most common form of treatment since the 1960's. They are uniquely effective and provide relief of symptoms in up to 80 percent of patients accurately diagnosed with ADHD.

Currently, there is a range of different short and long acting stimulant formulations.

The nonstimulant formulations have also become available in long acting formulations. The nonstimulants also provide effective relief of ADHD symptoms for many patients.

Two of the nonstimulants guanfacine and clonidine were used previously to treat hypertension. It was a welcome discovery that they also helped with ADHD.

STIMULANT
MEDICATIONS

There are two groups of stimulants used at this time for the treatment of ADHD.

1. Methylphenidate and its various formulations

2. Dextroamphetamine and its various formulations

Lisdexamfetamine (Vyvanse) is a newer medication that is converted into an amphetamine after it gets into the blood stream.

How   Stimulants
Work

Amphetamines and methylphenidate promote the release of catecholamines (primarily dopamine and norepinephrine) from their storage vesicles in the presynaptic nerve terminals and into the synaptic cleft. They also raise the levels of catecholamines by their ability to block the reuptake of norepinephrine and dopamine by competitive inhibition.

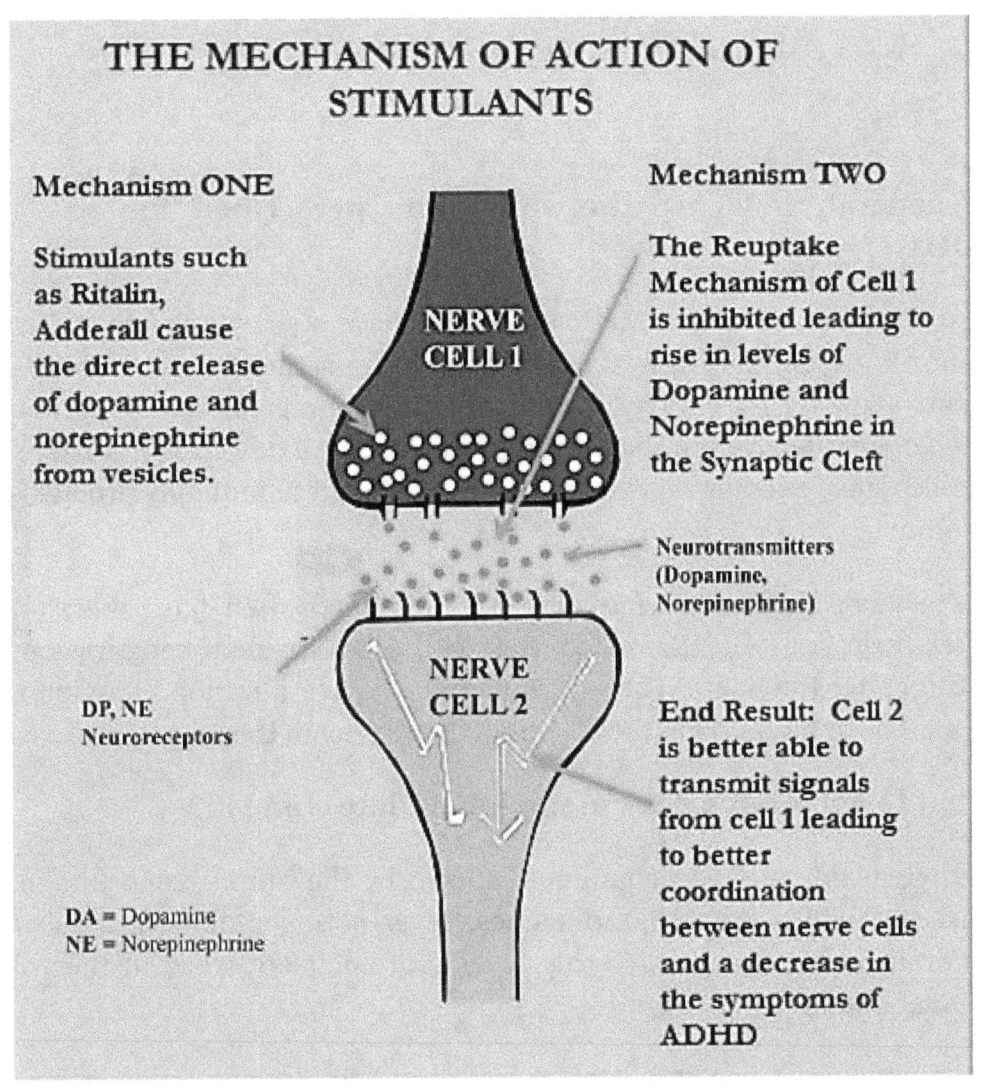

THE MECHANISM OF ACTION OF STIMULANTS

Mechanism ONE

Stimulants such as Ritalin, Adderall cause the direct release of dopamine and norepinephrine from vesicles.

NERVE CELL 1

Mechanism TWO

The Reuptake Mechanism of Cell 1 is inhibited leading to rise in levels of Dopamine and Norepinephrine in the Synaptic Cleft

Neurotransmitters (Dopamine, Norepinephrine)

NERVE CELL 2

DP, NE Neuroreceptors

End Result: Cell 2 is better able to transmit signals from cell 1 leading to better coordination between nerve cells and a decrease in the symptoms of ADHD

DA = Dopamine
NE = Norepinephrine

What clinical conditions are treated with stimulant medications?

There are three clinical situations where stimulant medications are the recommended treatment of choice. These are:

1. Narcolepsy

2. ADHD

3. Depression in elderly unable to tolerate other meds

In general, how are the stimulants prescribed for ADHD?

Dextroamphetamine and Methylphenidate have a short half-life and require administration 2 to 3 times a day. The longer acting formulations of these agents allow for once a day administration. The regular release formulation can be typically given in the morning, and a second dose is administered 4 to 6 hours later. Evening doses are generally avoided to limit any problems with insomnia.

The extended release formulation as mentioned often have the suffix SR (Slow Release), XR (Extended Release), XL(Extended Length), LA(Long Acting) after the name. These formulations have a duration of action that is about 8 to 10 hours. This allows once a day dosing in the morning.

What formulations does methylphenidate come in?

Methylphenidate is also commonly known by the brand name Ritalin. It is marketed under other brand names. It is not recommended for use in children under the age of 6 due to lack of adequate trials in the younger population.

Formulations: It comes as tablet, solution, slow release suspension, slow release capsules and as a dermal patch

Some of the extended release formulations are also available as generic extended release versions at a lower price than the brand name extended release formulations.

Here are the different brand names:

Ritalin (regular tablets come in 5, 10 and 20 mgs. The 20 mg is scored)

The tablets are chewable. The initial dose for children 6 years and older is 5 mgs by mouth twice a day before breakfast and lunch. The clinician may increase by 5 mgs at weekly intervals to titrate for effective response. It is available as a generic formulation.

Ritalin ER (It is dye fee and comes in 20 mgs strength)

Ritalin LA comes in 10, 20, 30, 40 mgs

(half is immediate release, half is extended release)

Metadate CD

It comes in 10, 20, 30, 40, 50 and 60 mgs capsule

(About one third is immediate release, about 2/3 is extended release)

Daytrana: This is a dermal patch that is applied to a fresh area of the skin daily for the first 9 hours of the day and then taken off. The effects last for about 3 hours after the patch is taken off.

It has the advantage of providing smooth levels through the day that are sustained into the evening hours to allow the child to finish their homework. It may also be useful in children who do not like to take oral tablets or capsules.

It comes in the following strengths

Daytrana 10mg, 15mg, 20mg and 30 mg patches.

Advantage: It can be useful in children that do not like to swallow tablets, or capsules.

A lower dosage is effective as the medication is absorbed directly into the blood stream and does not have to go through the first pass hepatic metabolism.

Quillivant XR

It comes as a powder for suspension. The strength is 25 mgs/5 ml

It comes in 60 ml, 120 ml, 150 ml and 180 ml containers.

Methylin

It comes as a solution of 5 mgs/5ml, 10 mg/5ml (500 ml dispenser)

It also comes as a chewable tablet of 2.5 mg, 5mg, and 10 mgs (scored) for children that have difficulty swallowing whole tablets.

(This formulation contains phenylalanine and should not be given to patients with phenylketonuria)

It also comes in tablet form in strengths of 5mg, 10 mg and 20 mgs it also comes as extended release tablet of 10 mgs, 20 mgs

Metadate ER Extended release version comes in 20 mgs strength

(Contains lactose, may be an issue in patients that are lactose intolerant even though the amount is small)

Concerta: This formulation looks like a capsule and has a cavity but is solid in appearance, does not dissolve and cannot be opened. It has a unique Osmotic-release oral system (OROS) MPH (Concerta). This involves a unique but simple mechanism. The extended release is achieved by expansion of a tissue behind a permeable osmotic barrier. As the osmotic saturation of the filling material occurs, it expands in volume and pushes the remaining medication through a small pinhole at the apex of the tablet.

Concerta comes in the following strengths: 18, 27, 36, and 54 mgs (slightly more than a third of the medication is immediate release while the rest is released slowly over 8 to 10 hours).

The Concerta tablet and other extended release products should be swallowed whole with water or other liquid and should not be chewed or cut. It may be taken with or without a meal. Concerta may have a duration of 10-12 hours. It is approved for both children, adolescents, and for adults

Dextro-MPH
(Focalin)

Available strengths: 2.5 mg, 5 mg, 10 mg tablet 4-6 hours' duration;

It is approved for children and adolescents.

Dextro-MPH XR

(Focalin XR)

Available strengths: 5 mg, 10 mg, 15mg, 20 mgs tablet. The duration of action is 8-10 hours. It is approved for children, adolescents, and adults. Focalin XR capsules can be opened and the beads may be mixed with applesauce or other food products if swallowing is a problem

Dextroamphetamine Formulations

Dextroamphetamine has been proven by clinical trials to be effective for the treatment of ADHD. It is considered safe for use in children younger than 6.

It is marketed under various brand names that are listed below.

Dexedrine, Dextrostat (It has 4-6 hours' duration of action and is approved for use in children and adolescents)

Tablets 5 mg and 10 mg

Dexedrine Spansule (Capsule, sustained release- It has 8 to 10 hour's duration and is approved for children and adolescents)

5 mg, 10 mg

Adderall, Adderall XR (Mixed Amphetamine Salts)

Mixed amphetamine salts (MAS) (Adderall) It has 4-6 hours' duration and is approved for children and adolescents

MAS extended release (Adderall XR) it has 8-10 hours' duration of action and is approved for children, adolescents, and adults

Dosages: 5mg, 10mg, 15mg, 20 mgs

Adderall XR capsules can be opened and the beads may be mixed with applesauce or other food products if swallowing is a problem.

ProCentra

(Oral solution is available as: 5 mg/5 mL (480 mL)
Tablet, oral as 5mgs and 10 mg

Dosing Guidelines

For ADHD

Oral: Children 3-5 years: Immediate release tablets or oral solution:

Initial: It is commonly prescribed with a low dose of 2.5 mg/day.

This may be increased at 2.5 mg/day increments once a week until therapeutic response is obtained,

The usual range usual range: 0.1-0.5 mg/kg/dose.

Children ≥6 years: Initial: 5 mg once or twice daily; may increase at 5 mg/day increments on a weekly interval basis until optimal response is reached, usual range: 0.1-0.5 mg/kg/dose (5-20 mg/day) (maximum dose: 40 mg/day)

Lisdexamfetamine (Vyvanse):

This is a unique prodrug compound that is inert until it is absorbed into the blood stream. There it is hydrolyzed (broken down) to the active compound of dextroamphetamine and inert compound L-lysine.

It is thought to have less of an abuse or diversion potential because of its lack of immediate pharmacological action.

It may have up to a 12-14 hours' duration of action. It is approved for children, adolescents, and adults.

Strengths are 20mgs, 30 mgs, 40 mgs, 50 mgs, 60 mgs, and 70 mgs

Its unique metabolism is illustrated below:

Vyvanse (Lisdexamfetamine) Mechanism of Action

Blood Vessel

PLASMA

RBC'S

RBC

Lisdexamfetamine

Hydrolytic Enzymes from RBC's

Dextroamphetamine

L-Lysine

Lisdexamfetamine is a prodrug that is acted upon by the hydrolytic enzymes in the blood stream to yield L-lysine and dextroamphetamine. The dextramphetamine is the active component that helps with ADHD. The original molecule Lisdexamfetamine is inactive and is less likely to be abused or diverted.

It therefore has a longer lag time before onset of action. This lack of immediate action is thought to lessen the risk and attraction for abuse.

Hypertension and stimulant use

If the person's blood pressure is controlled on current medications, it is relatively safe to utilize stimulant medications for ADHD. It would be prudent to obtain vitals at each follow-up visit while the treatment of ADHD is being adjusted. Another option for treatment is guanfacine, which can help with both the blood pressure and ADHD.

Why are immediate release products avoided in adults?

It is believed that immediate release products may lead to a more rapid rise in the level of stimulant medication. The rapid rise may cause a euphoric effect and thus increase the risk for misuse and addiction. The longer duration formulations have a more gradual rise and are less likely to be abused. This is however not felt to be a significant difference or concern with most individuals.

CONTRAINDICATIONS FOR STIMULANT USE

All stimulants should be avoided in patients who have structural heart defects, a history of recent stroke or heart attack, or uncontrolled hypertension. There is some baseline risk of sudden death in patients with these preexisting conditions and this risk may be elevated by stimulants.

All stimulants should be avoided in persons with paranoia, severe anxiety, hallucinations or agitation as these may be signs of a serious mental illness that can also be exacerbated by stimulant medications.

Stimulants should be avoided in persons with preexisting tic disorder. They can exacerbate the tics. Sometimes, new onset tics may occur during stimulant therapy. In these situations, the stimulant may be tapered off and a non-stimulant medication may be offered for treatment of ADHD.

Stimulants should be avoided by persons who have taken an MAOI inhibitor class of medication within the past 6 weeks.

Stimulants should not be used in persons who have any type of epilepsy as the stimulants may lower the seizure threshold and precipitate seizures.

They should also be avoided in persons with narrow angle glaucoma as dilation of the pupils by stimulants may exacerbate narrow angle glaucoma.

Stimulant medication should also be avoided in individuals who have been diagnosed with bipolar disorder, schizophrenia or schizoaffective disorder.

Stimulant medications may exacerbate these conditions.

It is important to monitor weight gain and height in children when they are prescribed stimulant medications. If there is a delay in weight gain or height gain, it may be prudent to lower the dose of the stimulant and monitor the appetite related side effects. Other strategies to deal with poor appetite are to offer more calories in the evening in way of larger meals and higher calorie snacks. The appetite suppressing effects of the stimulants wear off in the evenings when larger meals can overcome the poor intake at lunch. Another strategy is to provide drug holidays during seasonal holidays and summer break when the treatment of ADHD is not crucial to learning.

Stimulant medications should be avoided in pregnant women and those who are nursing infants.

If there are ongoing substance or alcohol abuse problems, the use of stimulants is also contraindicated. In these, situations, if there is a significant problem with ADHD or ADD after a full detox and medical stabilization, the non-stimulant medications such as guanfacine, atomoxetine, clonidine, desipramine, or venlafaxine may be more suitable options. Bupropion may also be considered, with the reminder or caveat that it cannot be used if there is a history of bulimia or of a seizure disorder.

Monitoring for Side effects

If an individual started on any stimulant medication experiences palpitations, feels anxious or notices any tics or skin picking problems, they should discontinue the stimulant medication.

The symptoms usually remit with stopping of the stimulant medication.

The clinician should monitor for appetite suppression or anorexia. One should also monitor the body weight and height of the growing child. An inquiry should be made about any symptoms related to insomnia or abnormal tics or movements. If there is an unusual increase in aggression or fluctuation of mood, it is prudent to discontinue the stimulant and seek alternative options for treatment of ADHD. Closer psychiatric monitoring is indicated until symptoms resolve.

If there is a problem related to insomnia, the dosage of any stimulant in the afternoon should be lowered or discontinued. In all cases of insomnia, sleep hygiene and the intake of caffeine should be reviewed. The use of clonidine, diphenhydramine or other sleep agents can be explored.

It is important to get the problem of insomnia under control as quickly as possible. Insomnia and lack of adequate rest compounds the attention and concentration problems.

COMMON SIDE EFFECTS FROM STIMULANT MEDS AND SOME SOLUTIONS

1. Insomnia

Solution:

Stop any evening dose of stimulant. Alternatively, go from the long acting to a short acting formulation.

Reduce caffeine intake in the evening. Any caffeine in the late afternoon can interfere with sleep onset and should be avoided.

Pay attention to sleep hygiene. Sleep hygiene is the set of bedtime rituals that either promote sleep or interfere with falling asleep.

Psychologically intense or disturbing shows on TV should be avoided before bedtime. Any video games of a similar nature should also be avoided at the hour of sleep.

A bath or shower, reading of a book, or listening to a book is generally conducive to sleep. Some individuals find a light snack around bedtime helpful for getting to sleep.

2. Nausea

Solution: Taking the medication with food may help to alleviate this.

3. *Anorexia or loss of appetite during mid day:*

Solutions: May increase food intake in the morning or evening when appetite is stronger.

4. Headaches

Solution: Headache can occur as a side effect with some ADHD medications. It can be triggered at the beginning of the dose of some ADHD medication such as bupropion, atomoxetine or stimulants.

Such withdrawal headaches can also occur when the medication is wearing off in the afternoon. Taking medication with food may slow absorption and help with morning headaches.

In the evening, if stimulant medications are used, a smaller short acting dose of the stimulant may help alleviate withdrawal related headaches in the afternoon. When headaches occur, vitals should be checked. If blood pressure is elevated, the medication should be changed.

5. Dry Mouth

Solution: Drinking extra fluids or using lozenges may help.

6. Dizziness

Solution: Lower dose and check blood pressure and vital signs. Rule out non medication related causes of dizziness. If it is due to the medication, consider change of medication.

7. Irritability and Mood changes

Solution: May need the dose to be adjusted down. If it is due to stimulant withdrawal in the afternoon, a shorter acting smaller dose of stimulant can be given in the afternoon to resolve the problem.

8. Tics

Solution: Lowering the dose of stimulant medication or replacing with a non-stimulant medication usually resolves the tic. Some literature indicates that ADHD patients have a higher rate for tic disorder even in the absence of stimulant use.

DANGEROUS INTERACTIONS BETWEEN MAOI ANTIDEPRESSANTS AND ADHD MEDICATIONS

Dopamine, serotonin, norepinephrine are small molecules that are discharged into the space between neurons to transmit messages from one neuron to another. They are called monoamines. Monoamine oxidase is the enzyme that rapidly breaks down these neurochemicals. By inhibiting this enzyme, these neurochemicals are not broken down and the levels of these neurochemicals rise.   If other medications are added that stimulate further release of these neurochemicals, the levels can rise to toxic levels.

The excess of dopamine and norepinephrine can be manifested by extreme hypertension, seizures, elevated body temperature, muscle spasms and toxic psychosis. The excess of serotonin causes a serotonin toxicity syndrome also known as the serotonin syndrome that is manifested by altered mental status, muscle fasciculation's, and unstable vital signs.

The MAOI medications cause enduring inhibition of enzymes that may last several weeks. It is vital therefore to no medications that enhance serotonin, dopamine or noradrenaline be used for at least 4 to 6 weeks after the last use of a MAOI agent. This will help to avoid an episode of malignant hypertension or a serotonin syndrome.

HOW SIGNIFICANT ARE THE RISKS OF METHAMPHETAMINE ABUSE AND DEPENDENCE IF PRESCRIBED FOR ADHD?

The risks of stimulant abuse are infrequent but not negligible. It is therefore important to be vigilant for any signs of abuse. In general, stimulants should not be prescribed for someone who has had a history of alcohol or drug abuse or anyone who has been convicted in the past for selling controlled substances.

The consensus however at this point amongst clinicians is that they are not abused by individuals who are properly diagnosed with ADHD. They are useful and effective and can make a significant difference.

Stimulants are useful meds in the right hands. They are used with great efficacy for some other conditions such as narcolepsy and certain refractory depressive states in the elderly. These depressive states in the elderly may be refractory to other antidepressants or the sideeffects maybe intolerable. Elderly depression can be marked by anergia (lack of energy), and anhedonia. Anhedonia is a bereft and humorless state of depression wherein the individual is unable to enjoy the things that gave them pleasure in the past. It is a pathological clinical state that can be accompanied by amotivation as well.

Some patients may misuse the medications and if this is found to be the case, the prescription should not be renewed. Some indications of an abusive pattern of prescription meds can be the asking for a refill because the patient lost the prescription or the medicine fell into the sink etc. If the patient starts losing their prescriptions or start seeking stimulants from more than one prescriber, the prescription of stimulant medications should be stopped. Some other manifestations of abusive use may be skin picking, severe dermatoses, insomnia, irritability, hyperactivity, and personality changes. The most severe manifestation of chronic amphetamine intoxication is psychosis. The risk of psychosis or mania is not present in the normal doses used to treat ADHD. It may however be a risk for those with underlying bipolar disorder or schizophrenia. In these conditions, the use of stimulants is contraindicated.

If there is any concern about misuse , the use of nonstimulant medications is always preferred for symptoms of ADHD.

NONSTIMULANT MEDICATIONS FOR ADHD

The FDA has approved the following non-stimulants for ADHD:

1. Atomoxetine (Straterra) It is used once a day and is gradually titrated up.

2. Clonidine modified release (Kapvay) The long acting form has a 12-hour duration of action. It can be used as an adjunct or by itself for the treatment of ADHD. It is more sedating than guanfacine.

3. Guanfacine extended release (Intuniv) Guanfacine has a long half- life duration and may range from 12 to 17 hours. The brand name Intuniv formulation has a duration of action of about 24 hours. It is effective as the sole therapy for ADHD in many patients. At other times, it is used as an adjunct to stimulant medications to help provide greater benefit for impulse control in addition to the beneficial effect on attention.

MECHANISM OF ACTION OF GUANFACINE AND CLONIDINE FOR ADHD

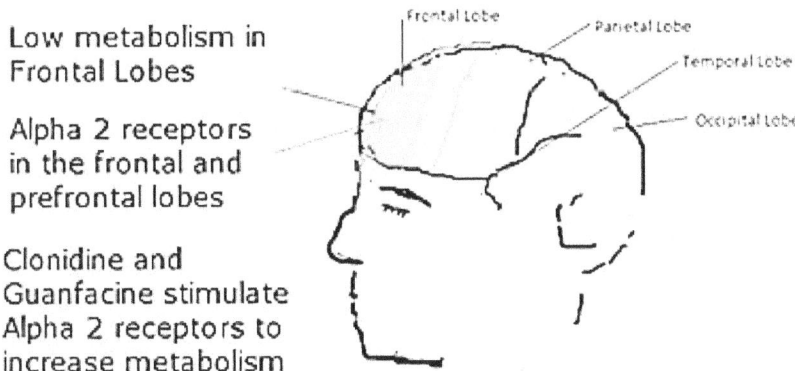

Low metabolism in Frontal Lobes

Alpha 2 receptors in the frontal and prefrontal lobes

Clonidine and Guanfacine stimulate Alpha 2 receptors to increase metabolism

Guanfacine has a more potent and more selective effect on the Alpha 2A subtype that is implicated in ADHD. Clonidine has broader effect on other Alpha 2 receptors and is thus more sedating.

There are five types of adrenergic receptors. Adrenergic receptors are those that when activated cause the release of stimulant neurotransmitter. There are two broad groups' alpha and beta. Among alpha, there are two subtypes α_1, α_2. Among the beta receptors, there are three main subtypes namely $\beta 1$, β_2, and β_3

Within these, there are further subtypes of receptors. Thus for example; the α_2 receptor has 3 subtypes: the α_{2A}, the α_{2B}, and α_{2C}

Clonidine stimulates all 3 subtypes of $\alpha_{2A, B \text{ and } C}$ receptors and thereby has more broad effects and greater side effect of sedation.

Guanfacine more selectively interacts with the α_{2A} subtype in the prefrontal lobe and is also a more potent agonist (stimulant) at this receptor than clonidine. By stimulating the postsynaptic alpha 2a (α_{2A}) receptors, guanfacine is thought to improves the prefrontal transmission of norepinephrine between neurons in the frontal lobe.

This may overcome some of the low metabolism in this brain area demonstrated in the Zametkin studies on ADHD.

Guanfacine for ADHD

Half Life is the amount of time in which half of the drug is excreted from the body.

Half-life for guanfacine is about 17 hours.

Indications

1.   ADHD

2.   Pervasive Developmental Disorder

3.   Hypertension

4.   Tic Disorders

Prescribing Guidelines for Guanfacine:

The initial dose may start at 0.5 mgs and be titrated up to 1 mg after 7 days. It may then be titrated up by 0.5 to 1 mg every 7 to 10 days and titrated for therapeutic response. The generic version is cheaper and has a relatively long half-life allowing it to be prescribed once a day or in two divided doses. A slow titration prevents side effects and improves compliance. The maximum dose is 3 mgs per day per the FDA guidelines for the regular release guanfacine.

The extended release (Intuniv) is approved as a treatment for ADHD in children older than 6 years and adults. It is usually prescribed once a day starting at 1 mg for the dose is titrated to response by increments of 1 mg every 4 to 7 days up to a total dose of 3 to 4 mgs. There may be less fluctuation of blood levels and a smoother and more extended response with the longer acting brand formulation.

If the patient skips or misses two or more consecutive doses, repeat titration up of the dose is recommended starting at 1 mg. If the patient is to be taken off the medication, a decrease of 1 mg per week is recommended to avoid rebound increase in heart rate or elevation of blood pressure.

Dosage Forms of Guanfacine

Generic Tablet guanfacine

Tablet, oral: 1 mg, 2 mg

Brand Name Tablet guanfacine- regular release, oral

Tenex®: 1 mg, 2 mg

Tablet, extended release guanfacine, oral

Intuniv®: 1 mg, 2 mg, 3 mg, 4 mg

What are some of the side effects of Guanfacine?

Side effects: Some of the following side effects may be experienced with guanfacine:

Headache, somnolence, fatigue, and dizziness, slowing of heart rate, decreased blood pressure, decrease of appetite, abdominal pain or discomfort. Giving with food may decrease side effects. Most side effects occur within the first 30 days. Slow titration may be helpful in limiting the side effects.

Food
Interactions

Extended release formulation: A high-fat meal increases peak concentration by 75% and AUC by 40% compared to the fasting state

Pregnancy Risk Factor

B (This means that animal studies have not demonstrated a risk to the fetus and data in human pregnancy is limited due to lack of studies)

Pregnancy
Implications

Some fetal risk indicated in animal studies. No data for human pregnancy exists. It is recommended that use during pregnancy should only occur if the benefits justify the risk to the fetus. There are no adequate and well-controlled studies in pregnant women.

.

Clonidine and its use in ADHD

Mechanism of Action:

As explained earlier, it like guanfacine is also a central alpha 2 agonist

Half Life is 12-16 hours

Maximum Dose: 0.4 mgs

Brand Names:

Kapvay®, Apo-Clonidine®;

Indications:

HTN ADHD

Chronic Pain

Tic disorders

Pervasive Developmental Disorders

Prescribing Guidelines

With Children <45 kg,

Initial dose

(0.05/kg) mgs per day split into two doses

May increase in 4 to 7 days if needed by 0.05 mgs/kg

Dose titration is started at the lowest dose of 0.1 mg half tab once or twice a day. A slow titration will avoid side effects of sedation or dizziness due to hypotension (decreased blood pressure).

Dosage Strengths and Formulations:

Clonidine comes as a patch and in regular and extended release tablet forms

Clonidine Patch, transdermal:

1. 0.1 mg/24 hours

2. 0.2 mg/24 hours

3. 0.3 mg/24 hours

The patch should be taken off if the person has to have a MRI scan for any reason. The patch has metal elements such as aluminum that is affected by the strong magnetic fields created during the MRI procedure.

Clonidine Tablet,

0.1 mg, 0.2 mg, 0.3 mg Catapres®: 0.1 mg, 0.2 mg, 0.3 mg [scored]

Tablet, extended release, oral, as hydrochloride: Kapvay®: 0.1 mg, 0.2 mg

Managing Side effects from Clonidine and Guanfacine

The following side effects are sometimes reported: sedation, fatigue, dizziness, mood changes, irritability, nightmares, localized skin reactions and some slowing of heart rate and lowering of blood pressure. Sexual dysfunction may occur in adults. These side effects do tend to decrease as the body adapts over time.

Sedation: The side effects of sedation tend to be greater with clonidine as compared to guanfacine. This side effect is utilized to help with insomnia by giving clonidine at bedtime.

If daytime drowsiness is a problem, the clinician may decrease the dose in half for one week to two weeks and go back up slowly if needed to better control ADHD symptoms.

Dizziness – The clinician can hold the dose and rule out any other causes of dizziness and treat those if present. The medication can be tried again with a slower titration schedule starting at a lower dose. If the patient is on other blood pressure medications, the dosage of these medications can be lowered.

The patient should be instructed to get up and arise slowly until symptoms resolve.

Sudden withdrawal should be avoided. Sudden withdrawal may be associated with rebound symptoms marked by increased heart rate and an elevation of blood pressure.

Bupropion (Wellbutrin, Zyban) for ADHD

Bupropion is an antidepressant and smoke cessation medication that has shown some efficacy with ADHD symptoms. It can be prescribed in the generic or the brand name form. For ADHD the Wellbutrin XL brand is useful as it can be dosed once in 24 hours. Bupropion (Wellbutrin, Zyban) is contraindicated in anyone with a history of seizures or bulimia. The dose can be started at Wellbutrin XL 150 mgs per day and this can be elevated to Wellbutrin XL 300 mgs once a day. The SR formulation dose can be used twice a day and should not exceed 200 mgs one time dose.

The regular generic bupropion should be started at 75 mgs one tab given twice a day and gradually titrated up to 150 mgs by mouth twice a day. The one time dose of regular release bupropion should not exceed 150 mgs. Higher one time doses may be associated with a greater risk for seizures.

Mechanism of Action:

This is not fully understood but is thought to be due to inhibition of the reuptake of dopamine and norepinephrine in the presynaptic neurons and thereby increasing the amount of dopamine and norepinephrine in the synaptic cleft.

Clinical Indications for bupropion (Wellbutrin, Zyban)

1. ADHD- this is an off label use and it is thought to be helpful for some ADHD patients

2. Depressive Syndromes: The advantage of using bupropion is the lack of sexual side effects that are often associated with other antidepressants belonging to the SSRI or Tricyclic antidepressant class.

3. Smoking Cessation - it has been shown to decrease cravings and raise the rates of abstinence from smoking.

Contraindications for Bupropion (Wellbutrin, Zyban):

Use is contraindicated in patients with seizure disorder or history of bulimia. It may lower the seizure threshold especially when the dosage goes above 300 mgs per day. The dosage for the immediate release version should not exceed 150 mgs, should not exceed 200 mgs for the SR version.

The dosage should be lowered to half in patients with mild to moderately impaired kidney function.

Side effects:

These include a small increase in heart rate, insomnia if given later in the day, weight loss, dry mouth, and nausea. Other side effects that may occur include headache, and dyspepsia. The long acting formulations are better tolerated than the immediate release formulations.

Formulations:

It comes in the following formulations

(Wellbutrin)

75 mgs and 100 mgs

150 mg

Tablet, 12-hour (Wellbutrin SR)

100 mg

150 mg

200 mg

Tablet, 12-hour (Zyban)

150 mg

Tablet, 24-hour (Budeprion XL, Wellbutrin XL)

150 mg

300 mg Tablets

Atomoxetine (Straterra) for ADHD

Atomoxetine is effective for some individuals with ADHD. It can have some side effects related to the gastrointestinal tract such as dyspepsia if the dose is titrated up too quickly. It is can be started at a low dose of 10 or 18 mgs and the dosage can be built up at weekly intervals. There may be a waiting period of 2 to 3 weeks before a therapeutic response is evident. In some individuals, the onset of benefits may be noticed sooner.

Available Strengths: It comes as a capsule in the following strengths:

10, 18, 25, 40, 60, 80 and 100 mgs capsules

Mechanism of Action:

It is a selective inhibitor of norepinephrine reuptake at the presynaptic neurons.

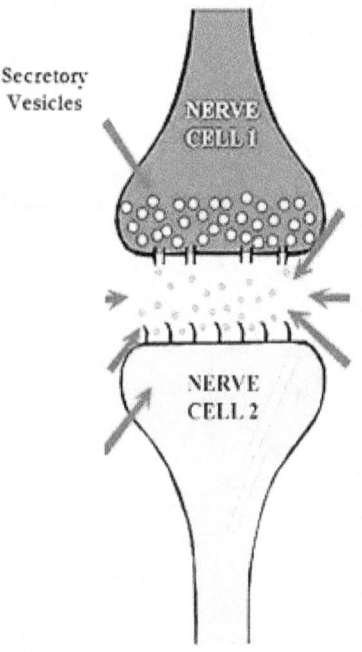

Atomoxetine (Straterra), Desipramine, Venlafaxine Mechanism of Action

Norepinephrine Re-Uptake Inhibited->>Norepinephrine Levels Increase->>ADHD Symptoms Decrease

Indications: It is indicated for ADHD

Data for use for children under six is limited and it is not recommended in this age group.

Precautions:

Atomoxetine belongs to a SNRI (Selective Norepinephrine Reuptake Inhibitor) class of medications. Medications belonging to the SSRI (Selective Serotonin Reuptake Inhibitor) or SNRI class have been linked in rare and infrequent cases to suicidal thinking in the first few weeks of treatment. Monitoring for such symptoms is indicated during the first few weeks of treatment.

It has also been linked with a rare and idiosyncratic hepatitis. If patients have yellowing of eyes or skin, itching, or flu like symptoms, the medications should be stopped and patient should be referred to a hospital for further workup and monitoring. The medication in this situation should stopped immediately. The liver function tests should be monitored. On rare occasions (2 cases) hepatotoxicity including hepatic failure may occur. The majority of cases occurred within the first 120 days, so that closer monitoring may be indicated during this time period.

Side effects: Some of the side effects may include dyspepsia, decreased appetite, abdominal pain, and sleep disturbance.

Pharmacokinetics: The half-life of atomoxetine is about 6 hours but it can be given once a day. Metabolism may vary between individuals significantly.

Atomoxetine should be avoided with CYP2D6 inhibitors to avoid elevation of levels of atomoxetine.

Dosage: 0.5 mgs/kg or even lower initially, and titrate up weekly by small increments

Titrate up slowly to avoid side effects while monitoring for patient acceptability and compliance by patient.

The treatment dose varies significantly for different patients

Dosage should not exceed 100 mgs in adults and should not exceed 80 mgs in children.

What are some guidelines in the treatment of ADHD with desipramine?

Noradrenergic tricyclic desipramine has been used to treat ADHD. The usual starting dose is 25 to 50 mgs and titration is done by 25 to 50 mgs every 4 to 7 days to limit side effects early on. The therapeutic dose is 150 to 200 mgs. Desipramine along with tricyclic antidepressants can have a wide variability in levels and can affect cardiac conduction. It is therefore a good idea to have a pretreatment EKG and a follow-up EKG once the patient has been stabilized. If the dose is ineffective, a blood level can be obtained, as some patients can be fast metabolizers. Desipramine should be avoided in anyone with cardiac disease.

Can Venlafaxine be used for ADHD?

Venlafaxine in doses above 150 mgs to 225 mgs has noradrenergic and dopaminergic actions. Some individuals have reported benefit for ADHD with this medication. It may cause a mild elevation of blood pressure in some individuals. Monitoring of blood pressure therefore is recommended. Venlafaxine, desipramine and other antidepressants should be used with caution in those with a history of bipolar disorder. This is because antidepressants can precipitate a relapse into mania.

VACATION FROM MEDICATIONS/ DISCONTINUING MEDS

A vacation from medications is possible as the child grows up and learns to manage symptoms in other ways. As the development of the brain continues into adolescence, the problems of inattention and hyperactivity may remit and get better.

Behavior therapy, cognitive retraining with cognitive behavioral therapy and learning of organizational skills may suffice for many individuals with ADHD.

Not all patients however go into remission of their ADHD by adulthood and a subset of patients require treatment through adolescence and adulthood.

Use of Antipsychotics

Generally speaking, the use of antipsychotics in children should be very infrequent, as they have no role in the treatment of ADHD. They may be useful sometimes with patients that have pervasive developmental disorder and associated aggressive behaviors with or without ADHD.

Chapter 6
Nonpharmacological   Strategies for ADHD

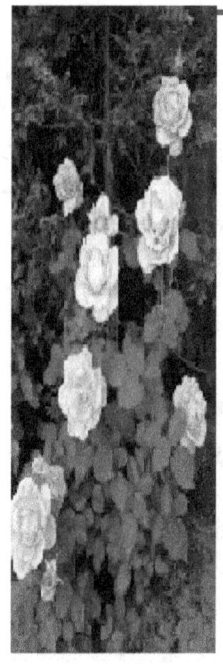

Organization training, Removing of Distractions

Neurofeedback

Transcendental Meditation, Other Meditation, Exercise

Removal from diet of Artificial Food Colors, Perservatives

CBT, Behavioral Therapy, ADHD Coaching

Alternative therapies are interventions other than medications that can be effectively used to treat symptoms of ADHD.

They can provide real and significant benefits for ADHD by decreasing symptoms with improved functioning.

Alternative therapies range from structuring the environment to limiting distractions. They may also involve altering dietary intake by removing artificial food colors and preservatives. There is a study published in Lancet indicting that the ingestion of certain food colorings is associated with symptoms of ADHD.

Some therapies work wonderfully for some, while for others they may not do very much.

With as diffuse a syndrome as ADHD, which has multiple etiologies, such a differential response to different interventions is to be expected. The individual with ADHD should try as many of the different techniques as possible and use what works best for him or her.

The benefits may need time to build up, so patience is a virtue when trying out some of these techniques. If something works, that strategy can be retained and used on a regular basis by making it part of the lifestyle of the individual.

BEHAVIORAL THERAPY

Behavior therapy is a form of therapy used mostly in children based on the idea that the behavior that is rewarded is likely to be repeated and behavior that is ignored and not rewarded gradually decreases or "extinguishes" itself. Behavior therapy is often combined with other techniques for optimal effects.

Below are some components of behavior therapy.

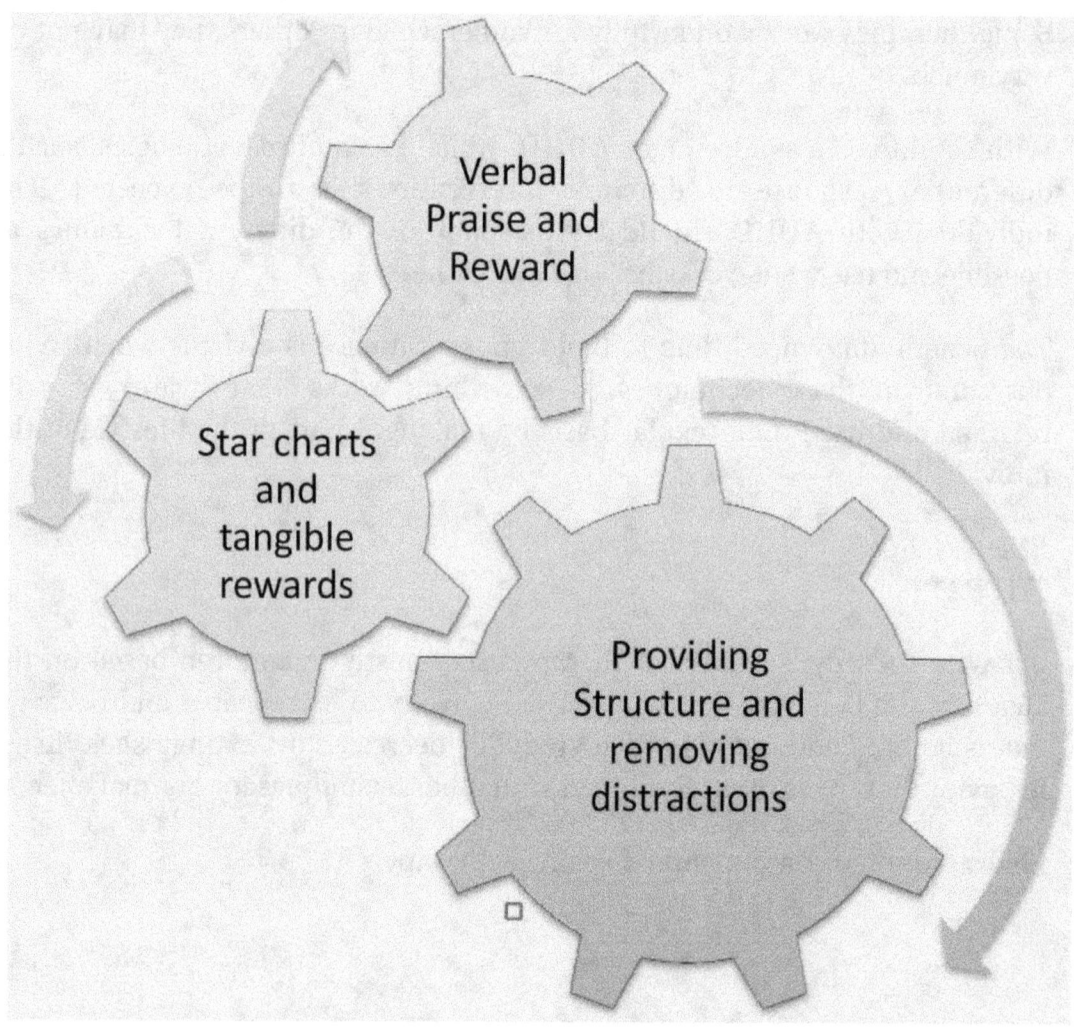

MODIFIYING DISRUPTIVE BEHAVIORS

Behavioral therapy can be used to mold and modify disruptive behaviors. Disruptive and intrusive behaviors are quite common with ADHD and can lead to suspension from school or legal problems. The specific behaviors that need to be changed are identified and a reward for a replacement behavior is chosen. In a systematic way, a plan can be created and implemented to change behaviors one step at a time.

Behavior therapy makes sense at an instinctual common sense level for most people. They easily understand the concept.

The key in any behavioral program however is consistency. A minor inconsistency can lead to an enduring relapse of undesirable behaviors.

A good behavioral therapist will try to "catch" the child doing something right and reward the child by verbal praise or some tangible reward. Examples of positive behaviors may be playing with others without fighting, sharing of toys with others or remembering to turn in classroom assignments on time.

Any improvement in these areas should be recognized by rewarded.

USING A COMBINATION OF TECHNIQUES

1. A list of desirable behaviors is made. The number of behaviors should be limited in number.

2. A list of rewards for desirable behaviors is made.

3. Star charts are set up to show progress towards a reward

4. A structured timetable is set up for play and work to provide structure

5. Work areas are prepared by removing distractions and noise

6. All directions are given in clear and simple language

7. Plan to be available to redirect and answer questions

8. Allow outdoor playtime in a safe environment of about 30 minutes whenever possible before study time. It helps to improve concentration.

9. One can participate in some activities and model behaviors.

10. A timer is used for "timeouts" to provide consistency for structuring length of activity or if time out is used.

11. The child can be praised in front of others for doing well

Avoid excessive criticism. Focus more on the positive.

Excessive criticism can make some children depressed with visible slouching and glum expression. Other children can express the depression through oppositional and defiant behaviors. It is important therefore to be realistic and not expect perfection. Any improvement should be acknowledged and clear guidance should be provided about expectations in a gentle and kind manner.

Learning and growth is best achieved in a tolerant supportive atmosphere where mistakes are not dwelled on and the focus remains on the positive gains made.

OTHER POINTS TO KEEP IN MIND

1. If medications and behavioral therapy are combined, it may be possible to use lower dosage of the medications.

2. The teaching of behavior management technique to parents and teachers is an important part of any behavioral treatment program.

3. This type of teaching allows everyone to be to be on the same page.

4. Such collaboration makes for consistency that is essential to the success of any behavioral treatment program.

5. One should be patient and supportive during behavior therapy and *never* get into a punitive stance.

6. Consistently apply the program by having set routines, removing distractions and rewarding on task performance.

STAR CHARTS ARE VERY USEFUL TOOLS- USE THEM

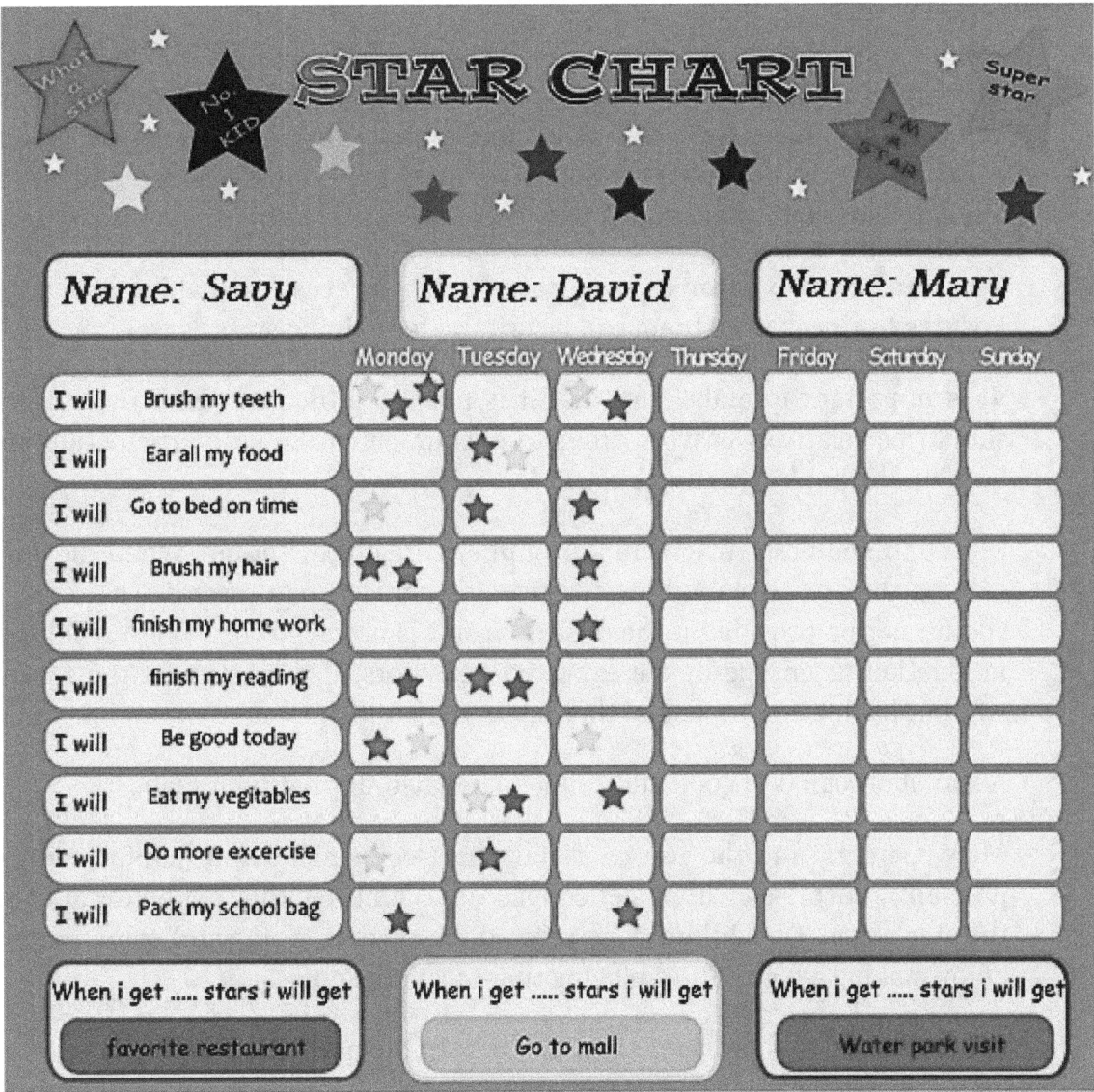

Star charts such as the one depicted above can be a very helpful tool for implementing behavioral therapy. The seeing of their progress in a visible and meritorious manner reinforces the desire of the child to do well.

Technique

The child is granted "their star" for performing a desired behavior such as "I will finish my reading" or "I will pack my school bag."

Other target behaviors where improvement is needed can be added to the list of behaviors. Each time the child performs as desired in regards to that behavior, he or she gets a reward. The stars are counted at the end of the week to figure out what reward they get.

Teachers can also become participants in this process of shaping behaviors. Positive feedback from them can be criteria for gaining stars as well.

It is important to make sure that it is not too difficult to earn the stars. It should be relatively easy in order to encourage continued participation and keep up the hope of getting a reward.

The chart should be placed in a prominent area of the home. When the child earns 5 stars or 10 stars, they are given an agreed upon reward. The rewards should not be provided if the desired result is not achieved. There will be no motivation to engage in the expected behaviors, if they still get the reward without having accomplished their expected number of stars or merits.

A star chart can be a good addition to a behavioral treatment plan.

Many parents find the use of a star chart convenient and helpful and are pleasantly surprised with it's effectiveness. With time, they get better at using the star chart. The child can be praised for earning a star and some parents enjoy making a big show of placing the star on the chart.

It can be a fun and pleasant exercise for both the parent and the child.

A Summary of Recommendations

- Behavior therapy is used to reinforce the desirable behaviors and to diminish the frequency of undesirable behaviors. Its basic tenants are as follows:

- Reinforce positive behaviors

- Have consequences for undesirable behaviors

- Remove distractions

- Structure time with a schedule that is predictable but not too busy

- Prepare work area by having tools for learning available such as pencils, erasers etc.

- Reward system is explained to the child and they are allowed to "buy into the program".

Earning the rewards and praise of others can build self-esteem and sense of competence in the child. When interventions are combined, a lower dosage of medications may suffice for control of ADHD symptoms.

What is the cognitive behavioral therapy (CBT) approach to ADHD?

CBT is used more commonly in adults. In this therapy, the main job of the therapist is to instill a sense of mastery in a person over the flow of their own thoughts. It teaches them to sort divergent thoughts in order to better sort out what is relevant to the task at hand.

The treatment is also geared towards removing cognitive blocks and distortions that prevent in gaining focus and attention.

Cognitive distortions are basically erroneous conclusions that a person has made about themselves and their world. These are examined together and the individual is trained to recognize them in daily life. They are encouraged to let go of the distortions and are encouraged to replace them with more logical and more empowering beliefs.

The distortions usually center around their ability to solve problems and their ability to become more organized. Their confidence in their ability to do this is low. It is the job of the therapist to show the distortions for what they are. When the distortions are removed, the individual gains the confidence in being able to achieve their goals. With renewed confidence they are able to use the knowledge they always had.

Through news ways of thinking about things with the help of CBT, individuals can turn their life around towards greater productivity and enhanced satisfaction with their lives.

COMMON DISTORTIONS

Not Enough Time:

One of the distortions in the mind of the ADHD individual is a sense of not having enough time.

This becomes an easy excuse for impulsive decision making that is common in the person with ADHD.

By understanding that there is enough time for well thought out decisions, impulsive and rash decisions can be avoided.

Clarifying this distortion leads to patience and deliberation before actions.

Hyperfocus

Another pattern is to hyperfocus on a few details and miss the larger picture.

Giving Up Too Fast

In this state of mind, the person is convinced that they cannot do better. They consequently give up on their efforts prematurely.

Self-Defeating Behaviors

Self-defeating behaviors tend to germinate in the gloom and repeated frustrations associated with ADHD.

The self-defeating behaviors listed below may crop up and try to sabotage the newfound success of the person. The job of the therapist is to encourage the person to adopt rational modes of thinking and to avoid the self-defeating behaviors.

Some self-defeating behaviors may take on the following forms.

- Avoidance

- Procrastination

- Working on multiple projects

- Resignation and Pessimism

- Nihilism

- Alcohol and drug use

- Distracting oneself by creating other problems

- Focusing on nonessential tasks

TM (TRANSCENDENTAL MEDITATION) FOR ADHD

A steady stream of encouraging testimonials have kept flowing in about the positive effects of TM since it was introduced to the world in 1955 by an Indian ascetic Maharishi Mahesh Yogi.

Studies about TM

Many studies about the physiological and neurological effects of TM have been completed over the last 40 years.

A listing of the studies substantiating benefits can be found at this website. http://wwv.tm.org/research.html

TM is not a hoax. There is something real and valuable going on with this technique.

SCIENTIFIC STUDIES DONE ON TM, COGNITIVE FUNCTION AND ADHD.

1. Gross Wald S, Stixrud W, Travis F, Bateh M. Use of the Transcendental Meditation technique to reduce symptoms of ADHD by reducing stress and anxiety Current Issues in Education, (2009), 10 (2) online.

2. So KT, Orme-Johnson DW, Three randomized experiments on the holistic longitudinal effects of the Transcendental Meditation technique on cognition. Intelligence (2001), 29 (5):419-440

3. Travis, F & Arenander, A Cross sectional and longitudinal study of the effects of transcendental meditation practice on inter-hemispheric frontal asymmetry and frontal coherence. International Journal of Psychophysiology (2006), 116: 1519-38.

4. Dillbeck, M.C., &Bronson, E.C. Short term longitudinal effects of the Transcendental Meditation technique on EEG power and coherence. International Journal of Neuroscience (1981) 14, 147-151

Books on Transcendental Meditation

Transcendence   by Norman Rosenthal MD

Catching the Big Fish: Meditation, Consciousness, and Creativity by David Lynch

Transcendental Meditation by Jack Forem

Symphony of Silence.   - An Enlightened Vision by George A Ellis

Celebrities and TM

Many celebrities such as the Beatles, Grateful Dead, Oprah, Jerry Seinfeld and Dr. Oz and his entire staff attest to the benefits of TM.

Clint Eastwood along with many other celebrities has provide positive feedback about his experience with TM. He has indicated that it helped him "to get things *done*." This is true for many others also who find their creativity and ability to finish projects increasing with the practice of TM.

Schools and TM

In Brazil, Mexico and several other countries, school programs to teach TM and to allow regular times for meditation have been implemented. Some pilot programs in the US have also been implemented.

Schools that have implemented it for their students have seen attendance go up and rates of delinquency and suspensions go down.

Finding a TM Teacher:

To find a teacher near you, you can call 1800LEARNTM

or go to http://www.tm.org

The Subtle Layers of Refined Consciousness

The below diagram illustrates the key processes involved in achieving a state of mind that has been linked to the many positive effects cited in the studies. The regular contact with more peaceful and settled states of mind has a pacifying effect on many other areas of a person's life.

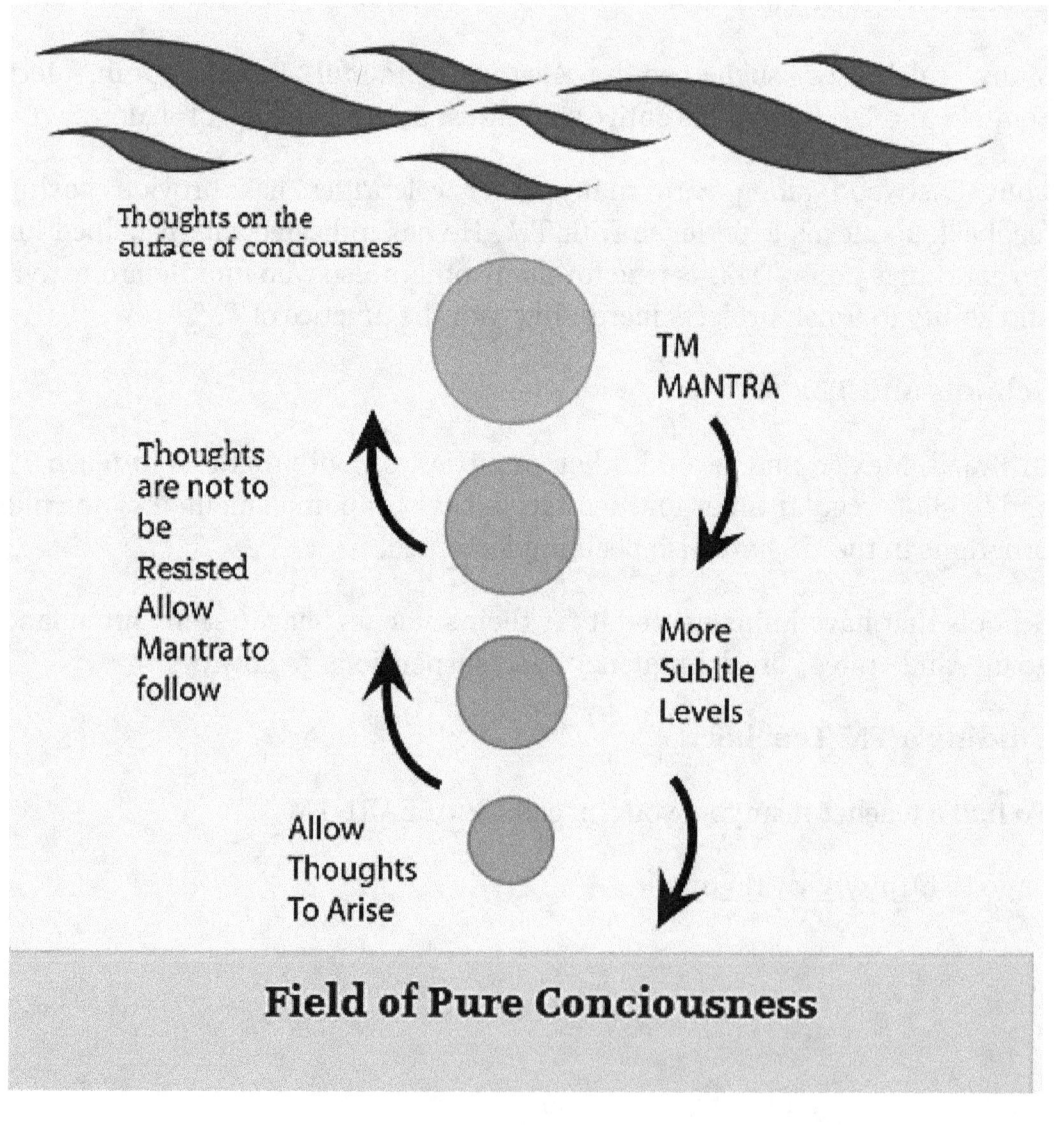

Thoughts on the surface of conciousness

TM MANTRA

Thoughts are not to be Resisted Allow Mantra to follow

More Subltle Levels

Allow Thoughts To Arise

Field of Pure Conciousness

How TM decreases symptoms of ADHD

There is an indication of increased frontal lobe and occipital lobe blood flow during TM according to a study done By Jevning et al.

This may be compensating for the corresponding decrease of frontal lobe metabolism in ADHD patients demonstrated in studies done by Zametkin et al.

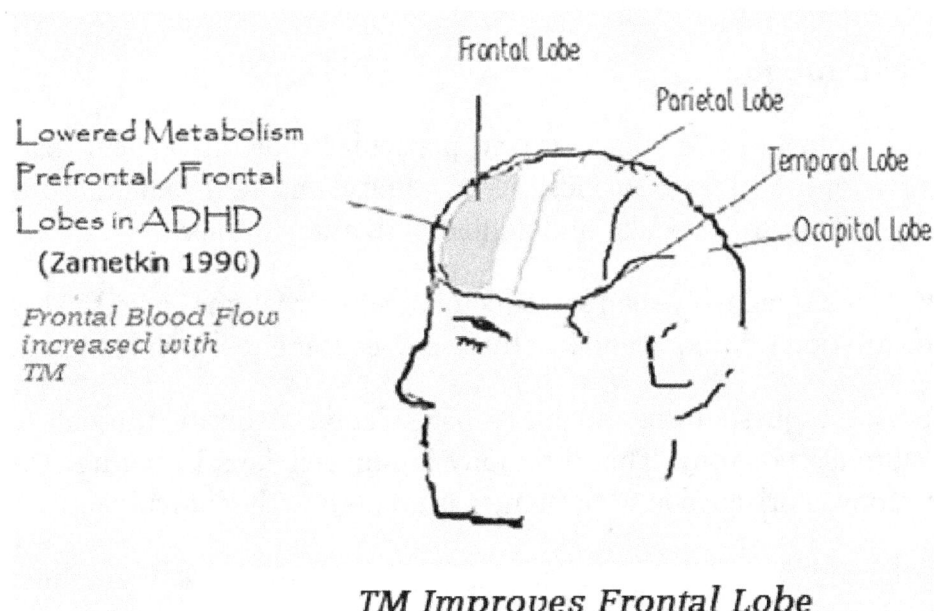

Lowered Metabolism
Prefrontal/Frontal
Lobes in ADHD
(Zametkin 1990)

Frontal Blood Flow increased with TM

Frontal Lobe

Parietal Lobe

Temporal Lobe

Occipital Lobe

TM Improves Frontal Lobe Blood Flow

Transcendental Meditation for ADHD has been shown to be useful in decreasing symptoms of ADHD by improving concentration and decision-making. It also helps with symptoms of hyperactivity.

Some interesting changes have been noted in EEG tracings of meditators. During meditation, greater coherence of brain wave patterns between different areas of the brain has been noted.

TM is reported to increase creativity, productivity and concentration. It also is noted to help with anxiety, depression, and other stress-related conditions.

The children who practice TM are reported to be less stressed and more focused. They also show improved grades subsequent to starting their TM practice.

In adults, TM leads to better planning, improved problem solving, and an improved ability to finish tasks through enhanced concentration and focus.

The TM Technique

In order to practice TM, there are no particular religious beliefs that one needs to adopt. You can, in fact, be an atheist and still benefit from the meditation. It is a truly secular and nondenominational practice.

The TM technique involves an introductory lecture that goes over the history of the meditation technique and briefly discusses some research behind it.

If the person requests to be taught Transcendental Meditation, a date is set for the formal ceremony. This ceremony is non-religious in nature. During the ceremony, a private sound or mantra is granted to the individual.

During the first lesson, the teacher meditates with the initiate and answers any questions from the new meditator.

A periodic checkup at 1 month and at any other time the meditator wishes is offered as a part of the course.

The technique is practiced twice a day for 20 minutes. The benefits for ADHD and for other areas of functioning are noticeable in a few weeks and months. They tend to accrue and consolidate over time. TM can become a great resource for coping with stress through the entire lifetime of the individual.

"Natural Environment" as a treatment for ADHD

A Potential Natural Treatment for Attention-Deficit/Hyperactivity Disorder: Evidence from a National Study Frances E. Kuo, PhD and Andrea Faber Taylor, *PhD*

According to the above study published in the National Journal of Public Health in 2004, it was found that allowing children to play in a natural setting for 30 minutes decreased the symptoms of ADHD.

This setting can be a park or playground where there are trees and a natural landscape with greenery and plants. Allowing play for 30 minutes in such settings can help them to stay focused for the next couple of hours with greater ease.

The theory is that ordinarily, there is "attention fatigue" with sustained attention in unnatural environments. Exposure to natural environments allows the mind to be freed from any effort to focus on the unnatural. This allows for a more rapid recovery of brain for continued cognitive effort.

In other words, natural environments are naturally calming and attention does not struggle to orient itself. This makes for less attention fatigue. Some individuals place plants in their office and find the presence calming and conducive to good attention and concentration. Having a window view of natural green scenery is said to have a more calming effect than the view of a concrete yard.

USING MODELS TO IMPROVE CONCENTRATION AND FOCUS!

The use of models can also help to build concentration when one is working on a project. Having an object representing the project or idea facilitates the continued focus and resumption of focus if interrupted. This facilitates the ultimate completion of the task.

Even NASA makes use of models when faced with tough problems. For those in other countries that do not know, NASA stands for National Aeronautics and Space Administration. It is part of the United States government and is the agency that helped put the first man on the moon.

When there was a crisis on the Apollo 13 mission, scientists resorted to models to solve the problem. This drama was reenacted in the movie starring Tom Hanks and named "Apollo 13."

During this mission, as the spaceship was on its way to the moon, there was an explosion in the main command module which housed the astronauts. This had compromised the power system and affected the ability of the module to regulate the internal atmosphere. The carbon dioxide levels in the cabin began to rise and time was of the essence.

In order to solve the problem, the scientists made a list of every object available to the Apollo 13 astronauts and placed the objects in an open area where they could be seen by all of the scientists. The scientists were then charged with the mission of coming up with a solution to fix the compromised the power system. Working against a deadline and using models, they were able to come up with a brilliant jury-rigged solution that dazzled the world and brought the spacefarers safely back home in the nick of time. This was a heroic accomplishment facilitated in no small measure by the use of models.

In the Mars Exploration Rover Mission (MER), the rover ran into some difficulties and began to malfunction. A similar strategy was used by having a life size model of the Mars Rover at the Jet Propulsion Laboratory in Pasadena. The scientists were able to manipulate the model and the electronics in any way they needed to come up with a solution. Having a real object in front of them greatly increased their ability to visualize and come up with ideas that ultimately solved the problem and fixed the rover for the next decade.

The point of these anecdotes is to drive home the point that creating models and using models can help greatly with focus and concentration. Individuals with ADHD can use models with great benefit when working towards a project or assignment.

EXPLORING WHAT WORKS

You should explore the different options that are available for treatment. Using one or more interventions together creates a synergy that enhances the effect of other treatments. The benefits of different treatments accrue and add up to an overall improved functioning of the individual.

Organizational tips can make a profound difference. Learning some simple methods can reduce the clutter in a person's life. Reducing clutter in the environment can create a climate that is conducive to good focus and concentration.

A healthy lifestyle that ensures an adequate amount of sleep and rest can improve the ability to focus and concentrate as well.

Avoiding toxic relationships can improve focus and concentration as well. If someone metaphorically gets under your skin or gets in your head, it can be hard to get focused. One must use techniques and coping skills to let go of the negative effects of the other person or persons. A lotus can still bloom though the waters be murky. One can learn to let the negativity roll off one's back and not let it affect the calm and focus. With calm and focus, corrective actions can be taken that are not possible in a state of distress.

Luminosity.Com website and app: This website has exercise that if done regularly for two to three weeks can help build focus and concentration. A mobile app is also available for mobile devices. This is an underutilized resource and can provide real benefits for some individuals with concentration problems. The exercises should be done for 5 to 10 minutes a day to achieve continued benefits.

What is known about neurofeedback therapy for ADHD?

Neurofeedback studies have shown benefit in the past but this was explained away or minimized. There is growing evidence from more recent studies that neurofeedback does indeed work for the treatment of ADHD. The change may not be dramatic as with medications but they are lasting and do not have the risk of side effects that some medicines may have. Neurofeedback is thus an important option to keep on the table for patients.

During neurofeedback, the person learns to produce brain waves that are associated with calm and focus. The data from EEG leads about brainwaves is fed into a computer that projects images on to a screen. The image for example may be of flowers of vibrant colors that bloom when the EEG is of a good focus state. When the mind is an unfocussed state, the flowers may begin to wilt and turn gray providing immediate visual feedback. The individual can learn to control the brain waves to keep the flowers looking fresh and vibrant in color. By such training, the individual is able to produce brain waves at will that are associated with good concentration for sustained periods.

Given the results from some of the positive studies, neurofeedback is a promising possibility in the future.

This fact may however get buried in corporatized medical journalism.

The clinician should maintain objectivity however and keep an open mind about using neurofeedback for individuals that prefer to avoid using medications to treat ADHD.

Are there products available in the market that can provide neurofeedback therapy?

There are various electronic products currently available that provide neurobiofeedback and can improve attention and concentration. They have become within the purchasing reach of ordinary citizens and the prices are expected to be even lower in the future. An example of such a product is below:

The Sony Complete SMART PlayStation One & and Play Station 2 System that prices at around 640 dollars. The Micrsoft X Box series is also compatible with software for bio feedback.

Other products are advertised on the Internet by different companies. This article explains the role of biofeedback machines and ADHD in further detail. It is posted at this website

http://www.playattention.com/play-attention-long/?

There are a number of devices available at this and other sites for a price ranging from a couple of hundred dollars to thousands of dollars. As long as the device is providing accurate feedback and control, it should be effective in helping with decreasing ADHD.

"A Little Play Attention Goes A Long Way"
Additude Magazine

http://www.additudemag.com/adhdblogs/19/10697.html?utm_source=eletter&utm_medium=email&utm_campaign=April

What is an ADHD Coach?

An ADHD coach is an individual trained in recognizing the difficulties of ADHD individuals and the unique challenges they face in organizing their lives and completing their projects. Their services of a coach are relatively inexpensive and can make a big difference for persons wanting to overcome their ADHD. The ADHD coach can provide support, encouragement, guidance and also render specific advice for overcoming persistent difficulties related to ADHD. They will encourage treatment compliance, keeping of appointments and use of cognitive skills that enhance productivity and achievement of goals.

Coaches can also help the person transition to a new lifestyle that may emerge when ADHD symptoms are controlled. There is a risk that the person may lapse into rationalizations and secondary noncompliance and slip into their old ways of dysfunction. The familiar always has an air of comfort, even when it is dysfunctional and harmful to the interests of the person. A coach can provide the objectivity that is needed to pull oneself out of such neurotic quicksand. They can help the individual stay on the path to greater self-actualization and a more fulfilled life.

It is possible to find out if a coach is available in your area by going to their website at www.ADHDcoaches.org

What are some common sense ways of treating ADHD without medications?

As discussed earlier, effective non-pharmacological options also exist and work very well for some people. Some of these interventions are pretty straightforward and driven by common sense such as getting adequate amount of rest and sleep. The ADHD child or adult may have difficulties slowing down in the evenings and falling asleep. Having a routine that allows for non-stimulating environment and paying attention to sleep hygiene or pre-sleep routines that are not stimulating can help in obtaining adequate sleep.

Mild hypnotics such as diphenhydramine or prescription hypnotics can be used as well if needed. Exercise and play activities during the day always help with sleep onset. Removing artificial dyes and preservative from food may help a subset of children and adults. Many diets in the past have been proposed. In general, the person with ADHD should avoid artificial food colors and preservative in the diet. A balanced natural diet that incorporates whole grains and complex carbs is reported to be helpful. Complex carbohydrates are obtained from whole grain, vegetables, nuts and fruits.

It is worth trying to see such as diet helps. Even if it helps to a small degree, it can make a big difference. If there is specific food allergy or intolerance, modifying the diet to avoid the offending food may help as well.

The possibility of neurofeedback and biofeedback for ADHD has been mentioned.

Games of coordination or activities that involve coordinated routines and balance may also benefit concentration and focus.

Exercises on the website luminosity.com may be helpful in improving memory and concentration.

Medical and psychosocial issues should always be explored during the diagnostic workup. The medical workup can lead to discovery of medical issues that may have a role in producing symptoms that can look like ADHD. When these medical conditions are treated, there can be a resultant improvement in the attention and concentration without the need of additional medications.

Whenever there are significant psychosocial stressors, they should be addressed through practical advice and problem solving with the help of social services, and therapists as needed.

The use of cognitive behavioral therapy can be very useful for such anxieties as well for ADHD in both children and adults.

Can you give more information about the psychotherapies available for adult ADD / ADHD?

Some of the following psychotherapies are available and have been found to be helpful in the treatment of ADHD.

Cognitive Behavioral Therapy: This was discussed earlier. It involves correcting any misperceptions and errors in thinking about their problems related to ADHD. Some ADHD patients have resorted to pessimistic thinking and hopelessness about being able to function better. The therapist can identify these false perceptions and give a realistic expectation of improvement. They can point out the possibility of change in the future. Other distortions are also confronted and corrected in a systematic, logical manner. Homework exercises that disprove the false beliefs are utilized to increase confidence in more positive life enhancing beliefs.

Metacognitive therapy combines cognitive behavior therapy with some training on organizational skills. It has also been proven to have lasting and useful effects.

Supportive Interpersonal Therapy: This can help with anxieties that are related to prior struggles, setbacks. These anxieties can create dysfunctional patterns of interacting with others and are also known as neurosis or neurotic disorders. They can cause difficulties in following treatment for ADHD and in the achievement of other goals. Interpersonal therapy can explore the motives and dynamics of a person's inner life that may need to be sorted out so that they don't come in the way of treatment.

Family Therapy and Marriage Therapy: Family therapy can be helpful in improving the ability of family members to understand each other better. Over the years, the partners and family members may have developed resentments due to the problems resulting from the dysfunction caused by ADHD. Family therapy can allow the family members to understand the dysfunction for what it is. This realization alone may clear the air of prior misunderstandings.

The treatment of ADHD is only one component of a relationship and other issues should also be explored and addressed. It is practical and wise for the family members to not overestimate the benefits of ADHD treatment in transforming the person.

It is reasonable however to remain hopeful that some positive change will result. The change also accrues over time. In family therapy, the clinician should be supportive. He or she can help the family navigate through this period of mutual adjustment.

Support Groups for ADHD: Mutual support groups are available in some cities and can be a source of support and motivation.

ADHD Coaching: The ADHD coach can help in setting goals and deadlines. The coach can also offer practical advice on how to persevere and stay focused until a task is completed.

Professional Organizers: A professional organizer can come and take a look at the patient's situation and give advice on how to organize their scattered office or home for a less cluttered and less disorganized life.

A Brief Summary of Salient Ideas

The following nonpharmacological strategies are often helpful for ADHD and in gaining a better focus. The person does not have to implement all the strategies at once but each one may have a role at different times.

1. Remove or minimize distractions in the environment. This may mean cutting out distracting sounds by turning off TV or radio.

2. Have the material needed for a task organized and in one place.

3. Create a quiet workspace area can help. Turn off the TV and mute the phones. Let it go to voice mail. Distraction by a phone call can set you back 20 to 30 minutes even if the conversation only lasts 5 minutes

4. Organizers can help. This may include paper calendars, reminders, smart phone apps, and Sticky Post It notes

5. Using models, diagrams, sketches, web diagrams to visually represent the subject that deserves your attention. It will sustain focus and concentration for a longer period of time.

6. Attention to diet may be helpful. Avoidance of artificial food colors, and use of complex carbohydrates such as legumes, pulses, nuts, and fruits may be helpful. Dairy products such as yogurt and honey have also been reported to be helpful with focus and concentration.

7. Caffeine in limited amount can help. An excessive amounts can create anxiety, dyspepsia or palpitations and is unhelpful.

8. Contact with natural settings has been shown to help.

9. Meditations, especially Transcendental Meditation (TM) can help

10. Aerobic exercise before a task has been shown to help.

11. Martial arts classes, dancing, sports or other activities that involve coordinated rhythmic actions that activate the cerebellum can help.

12. Soothing music may aid in focusing attention and improving concentration.

13. Healthy, nurturing relationships may alleviate stress. Stress has been noted to exacerbate ADHD symptoms

14. Individual Therapy for cognitive training may be helpful

15. Automating activities that can be automated can help in reducing the need for constant vigil elsewhere. This can lessen distraction.

16. Electronic devices can help stay organized may be useful.

17. Breaking a big task into manageable subtasks helps.

Training of parents: The parents can be taught skills to reinforce desirable behaviors in children and also to not to fall into power struggles with defiant and oppositional acting out behaviors. Rewards work better than punishment. The consistent application of a behavioral program can lessen anxiety and also help to decrease conduct problems. A genuine positive regard of the child should accompany all such interventions. Humans are very perceptive and a negative or judgmental attitude will sabotage the possibility of success.

How to Give Directions to a child with ADHD

- Obtain his or her attention by calling his/her name in a non-threatening way Be specific in your command

- Have a pleasant voice and use simple sentences.

OTHER POINTS

- Acknowledge and reward positive behaviors at variable intervals.

- Do not appear distressed by oppositional or defiant behaviors but have consequences that were explained earlier.

- Do not make the consequences excessive but just enough to get the message across.

- Be consistent.

- Never use physical punishment or consequences that could be physically harmful to the child. Never use words to berate or denigrate a child or anyone else.

- Do not become overwhelmed - get respite and time out for yourself if needed.

- Pay attention to your own wellbeing so that you can model wellness.

- Do not get caught up in minor behaviors. Do not over control.

Do ADHD diets work?

Removing food additives has been useful for some patients. Others have recommended getting adequate amounts of omega 3 in the diet as a useful intervention. The data on these interventions is limited and sparse, but does exist.

A well-designed British study published in a prominent journal Lancet offers the strongest evidence that some artificial colors and preservatives may exacerbate or cause ADHD symptoms.

The study is listed below.

"Food additives and hyperactive behaviour in 3-year-old and 8/9-year-old children in the community: a randomized, double-blinded, placebo-controlled trial

Donna McCann, Angelina Barrett, Alison Cooper, Debbie Crumpler, Lindy Dalen, Kate Grimshaw, Elizabeth Kitchin, Kris Lok, Lucy P. Orteous,

Emily Prince, Edmund Sonuga-Barke, John O Warner, Jim Stevenson."

Findings: This study found that the *addition of artificial colors and sodium benzoate preservative in the diet of children resulted in increased hyperactivity*. This effect was noted in 3 year olds as well as 8/9 year olds.

This experiment used 153 three-year-old children and 144 eight to nine year olds. It was a randomized, double-blinded, placebo-controlled, and had a crossover trial to test whether intake of artificial food color and additives (AFCA) affected childhood behavior.

There was a rush to find flaws with the study soon after's its publication and some later studies "could not duplicate" the results.

The issue has garnered some activism and there has been a campaign in the United States for the removal of artificial dyes such as Yellow #5,

#6 and some red dyes . Removing these dyes has been linked with a decrease in symptoms of ADHD.

It is worth mentioning that many of these additives are not allowed in foods in Europe, but are allowed in the United States.

Further information about such activism can be found at this link

http://www.npr.org/blogs/thesalt/2013/10/18/236221076/moms-petition-mars-to-remove-artificial-dyes-from-m-ms

Some individuals and groups have advocated special diets for ADHD. Some of these claims are based on questionable evidence. A person with ADHD can try them and see if it works for them even though rigorous studies in this area are sparse. Among the different recommendations some groups make are the use of more natural complex carbohydrate diets and avoidance of processed foods and carbohydrates.

Some individuals with specific food allergies are reported to do better when the allergen is removed from their diets. An example is sensitivity to glutens or mild lactose intolerance.

What is Parent Child Interaction Therapy?

Parent–Child Interaction Therapy (PCIT) is a therapy wherein parents are trained to work with their children in a manner that encourages more pro-social and decreases disruptive behaviors. There is a similar model wherein teachers are also trained to encourage prosocial behaviors. It uses a combination of different methods such as being more directive when needed, teaching basic behavioral therapy principles, and the use of play and other activities to improve bonding between the parents and children. One of the acronyms that is sometimes used to teach the parents some key concepts is called PRIDE. It stands for the following:

P – Praise

R – Reflect

I – Imitate

D – Describe

E – Enjoyment of experiences and celebrations of success

MORE ABOUT TEACHING TO CHILDREN WITH ADHD

Many good teachers naturally and by instinct grasp the finer points of teaching. Many are informed about ADHD and recognize that some children require repetition of the salient and key points during a lesson.

The great teacher does not hold the condition of the child against the child but tries to work around the deficit when it exists.

They may try to improve learning by limiting distractions and providing structure in the classroom. An example of limiting distractions might be to seat the child in front of the class where he is able to focus on the teacher and the blackboard.

Prolonged lectures are avoided. Instead, the teacher interrupts himself to provide an anecdote or ask an interesting question related to the topic at hand.

Inattention becomes more evident when sustained effort is required for listening. The best teachers know how to summarize what they are saying periodically during the lecture as they delve deeper into the lesson.

The act of providing a summary helps the ADHD child or adult to stay oriented to the task at hand and relate the subsequent material to knowledge already learned.

The use of multiple modalities such as video, audio, or discussion, can facilitate learning.

By breaking the monotony of a lecture in such a way, the interest of the student's interest can be sustained for a longer period of time and the disability of ADHD can be overcome.

Another example of creative teaching sometimes may be to invite feedback from the students through their questions, show slides or pictures of the object under discussion, and have a discussion. At other times an amusing story, an experiment or a hands on model may get the point across better. Short video clips of the subject under discussion can enrich the discussion. Such videos are becoming more available on popular websites such as You Tube and may be worth exploring.

A good teacher can play a very significant role in the life of the child. The child's good qualities can be recognized and avenues can be given for them to express themselves further in their recognized fields of strength. Appropriate counseling and guidance towards appropriate careers that work well with ADHD is important information to share with the person that has ADHD. The parent or guardian should also be provided such information.

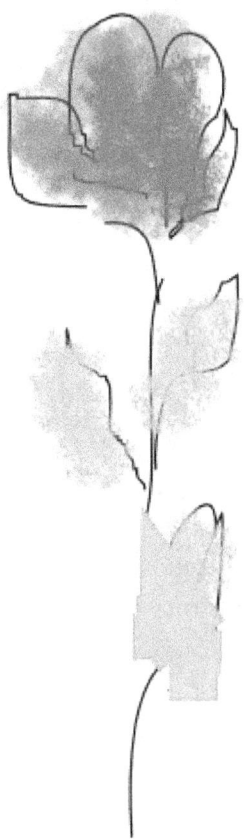

"Work with whatever tools you may have at your command, and better tools will be found as you go along." Napoleon Hill

Chapter 7
STRATEGIES TO STAY ORGANIZED

Getting it Together

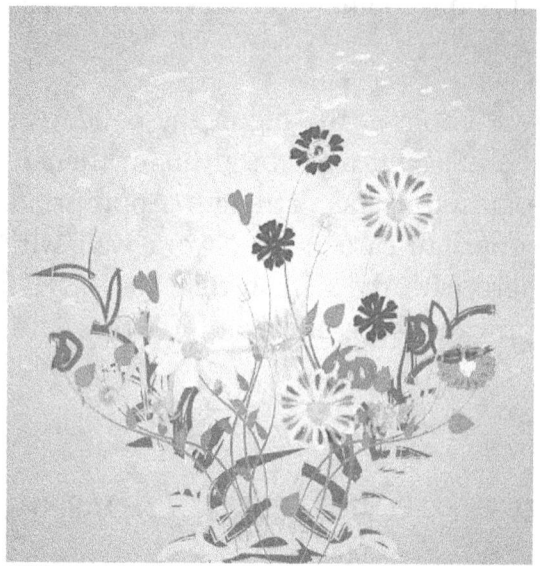

The following strategies can help one stay organized. You may use one or more of these strategies to gain control over your life.

OHIO technique for paperwork

- "Only handle it once" and make a decision about what to do with it.

- Make a decision about the paperwork as early as possible.

When you buy something, see if similar item that is no longer in use can be donated or thrown away so that objects not used don't add to the clutter.

- Cancel paper or unnecessary mail

- Request to stop junk mail

- Organize handbags or wallets once a week

- Put personal use items in one bag

- Declutter your closet- give away clothes you don't use

- Organize clothing by type

- Toss out extra wire hangers, give for recycling

- Store away winter clothes safely so that they are out of the way in the summer.

- Get socks of just two colors to avoid matching issues. Find the organizational hot spots; look at which area is the most disorganized? What is the most difficult to locate and designate a specific spot for it.

- Set deadlines for cleaning and decluttering your home

- Set a definite place for everything

- Set keys on hooks in one place

- Find" a home" for your different items and keep them at the same place

- Keep auto registration, license, and insurance in one place

- Recognize self-sabotage strategies and stop doing them. Some examples include taking on too much, not taking on enough, delay, procrastination, obsessing over unimportant details, getting into meaningless conflict, claiming something "urgent" has come up, losing supplies, forgetting passwords, failure to file paperwork in time, not checking on important mail, email, leaving things undone or partially done, reawakening toxic relationships you know are no good for you, being a glutton for punishment and wallowing in it. Take a minute to reflect on what you are doing and why you are doing it. If it does not add to your current goals, let it go and file it for later review. Set a goal and stick with it till you finish it. Not setting specific time bound goals can be a self-sabotage strategy to ensure the coveted success of the neurotic part of your personality. Use the deadline to drive your efforts.

Set a deadline for all your tasks and try to meet it. Schedule time to celebrate your success. Not celebrating your own success can be another self-sabotage strategy to take away the inspiration for future goals. Being excessively self-effacing is the same strategy with a different mask.

- The unfocussed semi competence of ADHD fosters self-sabotage due to frustration and soon it become a habit. When treatment of ADHD is pursued, letting go of these learned unhealthy behaviors becomes easier. If self-defeating habits do not improve, individual therapy may help the individual figure out what demons are they are trying to avoid by courting failure.

- Find a way to make yourself succeed instead of fail. Resolve to keep moving forward towards success even if it is by inches.

Preparing for success may involve the following:

1. Prepare for the next day

2. Check yourself before you leave your home, your car, your office or place you visit to see if you have everything and are not forgetting some article.

3. Don't carry sensitive items around that could be misplaced

4. Get a key chain if the loss of keys would cause a significant problem or security issue

Manage your time by

1. Keep a planner

2. Keep a small notebook for your to do list, stick with it

3. Have a list for work and go back to it at least twice a day keep oriented and on task with your priority task. ADHD individuals are masters at getting distracted and avoiding the list.

4. Avoid overscheduling

5. Delegate when possible

6. Find the time of day that works best for you

7. Early morning tends to work well with most ADHD patients

8. ***The telephone is for your convenience, and should not dictate your time.*** Put it on mute and pick up messages later when if you are working on an important assignment.

9. Learn skills to say no to interruptions

10. When interrupted by a nonurgent telephone call, end it soon by saying: "I have to get back to something, may I call you later?"

11. Set a time to return calls

    • Have scheduled routines to help you stay organized.

    • Make organizing and cleaning a meditation to relax, think and become calmer.

    • Teach your children organization skills.

    • Focus on one chore at a time.

    • Offer encouragement and support to yourself and others.

    • Use alarms and timers that are often available on smart phones. Allow yourself enough time.

    • Using a head set sometimes helps if you have to make frequent phone calls.

- If you need to call for service call companies at off peak hours, early or late in the day.

- Make a list of things to ask so that you don't forget.

- Use email productively and keeps email messages short.

- If you do not need a response, say so.

- Unsubscribe from mass mailings.

- Schedule a time to answer important emails.

- If you receive an attachment you are not expecting, do not open it impulsively.

- Send yourself an email for the important tasks for the next day.

- Figure out your most productive time and utilize it.

- Early mornings and midafternoons might be more productive for some individuals. For others late evenings and late nights work better.

- Do not try to be perfect. Let good enough be good enough if something nonessential is taking too much time.

- Avoid procrastination- don't over prepare.

- Look at events for the day, week, month, and set up reminders for a day before and an hour before. There are apps such as "Alarms" that are free or can be downloaded for a small charge to your cell phone.

- Use one main calendar to schedule everything if possible. The use of cloud technology may make this easier by coordinating scheduled events to be noted on a common calendar between the different devices.

- Allow for small breaks for rest and to remain productive.

- Just get into your project and start it and take one step at a time .

- Use automated bill pay when possible.

- Go to stores with a list

- Invest in money management software such as Quicken and others. Hire someone to do your taxes.

- Use direct deposit when possible

- Have a place for your bills.

- Have a box for receipts.

- Try "neat desk" software if possible.

- Reduce credit card use.

- Try to stay debt free.

- Have an emergency fund and plan your finances with the help of a financial planner.

- Consider reading book by Tony Robbins titled "Money – Mastering the Game". It has much advice that is precious for anyone but especially so for the person with ADHD.

- Take care of yourself physically, emotionally, spiritually; body, mind and spirit.

- Use meditation to heal yourself, and to promote organization and concentration.

- Engage in walking, exercise- it is good for you and the exercise helps with concentration during the day.

- Use models, drawings, and inanimate objects to represent your ideas or projects to help increase focus. The concrete representation helps to facilitate planning and sorting of ideas related to a project.

- Eat thoughtfully and not unthinkingly or on impulse.

- Avoid interactions with people that make you emotionally upset.

- Get enough sleep.

- Take power naps or a light siesta at midday if possible. It can significantly improve concentration and focus.

- Practice good sleep hygiene.

- Use meditations such as TM to center the mind to improve concentration.

- Develop your faith. It makes for a more settled and calmer existence and that always helps with focus and concentration.

- Have leisure activities that help you relax.

- Find a job that helps you and works well with ADHD.

- Leave yourself voice mails about what is to be done the next day.

- You can send emails to yourself in the future to remind yourself of something significant on that day or time.

  The website for this is at

  http://emailfuture. com/

- Use your creativity to come up with other solutions. There are many other ways to be more productive. Meditate on it and trust your imagination. Do not engage in anything that is illegal.

WHAT ARE SOME OTHER PRACTICAL METHODS AND WAYS TO LESSEN THE DYSFUNCTION CAUSED BY ADHD?

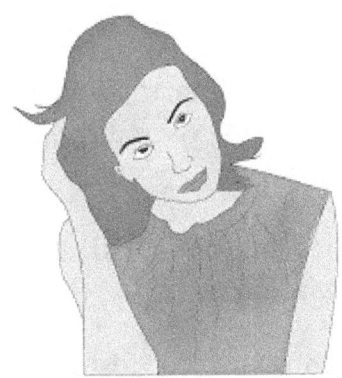

At the risk of some repetition, one can take one or more of the steps listed below to improve functioning.

1. Organize for the next day the night before.

2. Use of caffeine or tea by some adults with ADHD in the morning may be helpful.

3. Break up the task into smaller subtasks and reward yourself for achievement of each one.

4. Try to communicate with your supervisor at work if the climate is accepting of ADHD related disability. Federal law recognizes ADHD as a disability and discrimination for this on-the-job is unlawful.

5. Sometimes ADHD coaches may be of benefit.

6. Define and set goals and deadlines.

7.   Consider medication for ADHD and take them as prescribed.

8.   Recognize the time of day when you are able to focus and concentrate more easily. Use that time for your most important work.

     Most people work better in the mornings, whereas others tend to work better in the evening or late at night. Such patterns may change but are usually stable and it is useful to schedule yourself accordingly. During the designated work period, takes steps to avoid interruptions such as putting the phone on mute, turning off the TV or radio and even putting up a DO NOT DISTURB sign.

9.   Flexibility and choice are very helpful in getting the ADHD person to choose and focus on the things that they're interested in.

10. Go to ADHDsupport.com/teacher and attempt to foster a joint partnership with the teacher through communication and feedback. Become an advocate for your child.

11. It is helpful to have structure and to try to follow the same routine every day.

12. Post the schedule in big letters in a place where it is prominent.

13. Make time to organize for tomorrow

14. Set a location or home for everything such as your keys, your wallet and other items you utilize every day.

15. Simplify your wardrobe.

16. Spend about 15 minutes daily on decreasing your clutter.

17. Get enough sleep.

18. Take a power nap at midday if possible.

19. Get adequate exercise.

20. Get a complete history and physical done to make sure there are no medical issues that could be contributing to poor attention and impulsivity.

21. Having soothing music may help some people with their concentration.

22. Set a specific deadline for getting things done.

23. Get a consultation for ADHD related issues and take medication as prescribed.

24. Go for simple but elegant strategies.

25. Have only two colors of socks, black and white or black and brown so that a pair can always be found.

26. Use hooks instead of hangers if that helps.

27. Have trashcans in multiple places so that trash does not become clutter.

28. Start the day with a cleaning and organizing ritual.

29. Learn organizational skills.

30. Learn Yoga.

31. Learn Meditation such as Transcendental Meditation.

32. Join a martial arts class if possible

33. Use exercises that involve balancing or coordination so that the cerebellum of the brain (involved in such coordination) is stimulated. It gets better at coordinating thoughts through such activity.

34. Break big jobs into smaller tasks and set a deadline for the smaller tasks.

35. Get a recording machine to note your ideas; to do lists- most smart phones have this function.

36. Get iron free shirts and slacks.

37. Get electronic bill pay.

38. Have others help you, keep your workstation organized.

39. Get away from toxic people.

40. Read the section on how to use smart phones to increase your productivity.

41. Download some of the apps mentioned later in a subsequent section. These apps can help with productivity. You don't need to purchase all of them, only the ones that work for your needs.

42. Start the day with a cleaning and organizing ritual.

43. Learn organizational skills and meditation.

44. Learn how to use of timers, reminders and alarms.

45. Learn to set reasonable deadlines.

46. Have others help you keep your workstation organized.

47. Avoid conflicts that generate anxiety or distress.

CAN MUSIC HELP WITH ADHD?

Music that has a rhythmic light beat a soothing melody can help one focus and concentrate.

Different types of music help different persons. If a certain music works for you, use it on a repeated basis. Have more than one piece so you can rotate them. Sometimes no music and just silence is the best melody.

Some individuals report that Baroque music by artists such as Bach, Haydn, Mozart is helpful.

Baroque music has a unique cadence of 60 beats per minute that is in tune with a slow resting heart rate. The brain entrains itself to this rhythm and naturally falls into a relaxed yet focused state.

Incidentally, Baroque music composed during the Baroque era (1600 - 1750) has also been reported to be helpful for anxiety symptoms. You can get some more information about this at this website. http://www.anxaid.com/baroque_music.html#.VDoIzPnF-So

HOW CAN A PERSON USE THEIR SMART PHONE TO HELP WITH ADHD RELATED ISSUES?

This is a good question. Modern day smart phones have incredible amount of memory that can be used to store notes, addresses, pictures and videos in addition to just telephone numbers and email addresses. One can store calendars, alarms and reminders that can help a person with ADHD lead more organized and productive lives. Many people use the smart phones creatively in their own unique ways and for their own specific needs. They can be especially useful for someone with ADHD.

As an example, some of the following uses may be explored.

a)   Storing grocery lists

b)   Store to do lists

c)   Note where you placed something or where you parked your car. You can also take a picture of the area if you have a camera in the phone.

d)   Note clothing, ring sizes

e)   Jot down passwords. There is a password storage app called Password. It can help store passwords.

f)   Store driving directions

g)   Alarms can be set at preset times to alert for taking medications, make a call, attend a meeting etc.

h)   eBooks can be downloaded that may be audio or electronic reading format. The fonts may be adjustable for those that need to make them bigger.

i)   You can note ideas for a meeting or for work projects for the next day.

j)   An audio dictation app can be downloaded that can turn voice into text or store audio files detailing plans and ideas. Some examples may be the dragon app that is free or others such as Active Voice. The transcribed notes can be then uploaded and sent to email, Twitter or Facebook accounts or to a blog the person may have set up. New apps keep coming into the market that are remarkable and excellent. Pick one and stick with it.

k)   Keep track of new contacts by recording their details in audio or other format.

l)   The smart phone can also work as cd or MP 3 player that is able to store a good amount of your favorite music that may facilitate concentration and productivity.

m)   One can take a picture of an object or item that one wants to remember or even a picture of a page of to do lists that can be put as screens on the phone or sent as email to one's office for follow-up later.

WHAT ARE SOME SMART PHONE APPS THAT MAY HELP WITH ADHD?

Smart phones are becoming commonplace and can be a tremendous boon for keeping track of appointments, to do lists, but can also become a source of distraction. Having said that, the following apps are currently in the market that can in keeping information organized. The person with ADHD may find them very convenient and helpful. The phones and the apps be useful in organizing data and in planning. There is a tremendous creativity in this area among software writers and better apps are coming along all the time. They are relatively inexpensive or free. Here are some apps that have been found to be useful.

Epic
Win

It has a video gaming element that promotes sustained focus.

Task
Timer

It is a timer that tracks your progress. You can adjust it to your goals.

IReward Chart

It functions like a star chart wherein the child can visually see his progress with the number of stars.

Evernote You can store notes, audio, video, pictures and search for them easily later on. Many people love this app. A business version is available.

Dragon
Dictation

It works well to create speech to text documents.

B
e
n
t
o

This is a useful for storing different categories of data. The database is searchable and helps to decrease the clutter in the office.

Brain Trainer

This is an app created by Luminosity. It can help with increasing working memory and does improve the ability to stay on task.

FORGET

This app helps you to recall data that you may forget but can be triggered by keywords that are linked to the original data.

Dropbox

This is a useful information storage app. It is free and very useful.

Mindnode

This is useful for recording thoughts and ideas that may be otherwise lost if not recorded. It is reported to help with creative projects.

WHAT ARE THE TOP DISTRACTIONS AND WHAT CAN ONE DO TO MINIMIZE THEIR EFFECTS ON FOCUS AND CONCENTRATION?

The top distractions are reported to be as follows: Social Media - avoid logging on while you are at work.

TV- Enough said.

Email overload - set aside specific times of the day to take care of email. Cancel or unsubscribe from junk email.

On your cell phone - use caller ID and let it go to voice mail if you are busy.

When working, silence your phone.

Listen to voice mails at a preset time. Checking twice a day at mid-day and an hour or two before the end of the day should suffice.

Multitasking –This creates an illusion of getting more things done but studies have indicated that the person may actually be less effective when doing multitasking. Decide instead to prioritize and focus on one thing at a time until it is done and complete.

Boredom in ADHD - make a deal with yourself. Let it be that if you stay on task for 30 to 40 minutes, you get to take a 10 minute break and choose a reward. Have a timer or something to let you know it is time to get back to work.

Nagging thoughts - Write down what worries you. Take time to address them at a later date.

Go over what is important to you and remind yourself of your priorities and what's important to you so that the minor crises of the day do not overwhelm you.

Fatigue as a distraction: It is important to get a complete physical exam with laboratory exam as indicated to rule out any medical causes of fatigue. All the medications should also be reviewed as some can have fatigue and weakness as a side effect. If the person is medically sound, any psychiatric causes such as depression should also be ruled out.

If all is medically and psychiatrically well, the best way to overcome a feeling of fatigue is to get an adequate amount of sleep. For most, this is 6 to 8 hours per night. For some individual, a 30 minute power nap can help a great deal in boosting energy levels.

Meditation such as TM helps as well. Meditation such as TM for 15 to 20 minutes is said to be equal to provide deep rest and have the rejuvenating power equal to a cup of coffee.

Counterintuitively, sometimes exercise can help to overcome fatigue.

Hunger as a distraction: Have something light for breakfast or late breakfast. Try to not skip the morning meal.

Prefer fruit or high protein snacks when possible.

Choose complex carbs such as legumes, fruits and vegetables.

More about Depression - if you feel empty, hopeless, or indifferent-talk with a doctor or counselor. Treatment by psychotherapy with or without meds can be very helpful. The key to overcoming depression is to realize that you are never totally helpless. You can always control your thoughts and your perception of events and can put a positive spin on it. There is a silver lining to every cloud. Another fact is that you can always do something in your environment to make a difference. Exercising even a little bit of control over your circumstances can help to lift mood and decrease depression.

More About Medication - Check with the doctor if your medication or a known or unknown medical condition could be causing problems with your focus and concentration. Some medications such as topiramate (Topamax) may cause cognitive dulling directly or through elevation of ammonia levels. Some medications with anticholinergic properties may occasionally cause memory and concentration problems in some individuals. Such medications also often cause other side effects such as dry mouth, blurred vision, constipation and urinary hesitancy. High doses of of anticholinergic medications can result in an anticholinergic delirium especially in the elderly.

SOME SOLUTIONS FOR ADULT ADHD

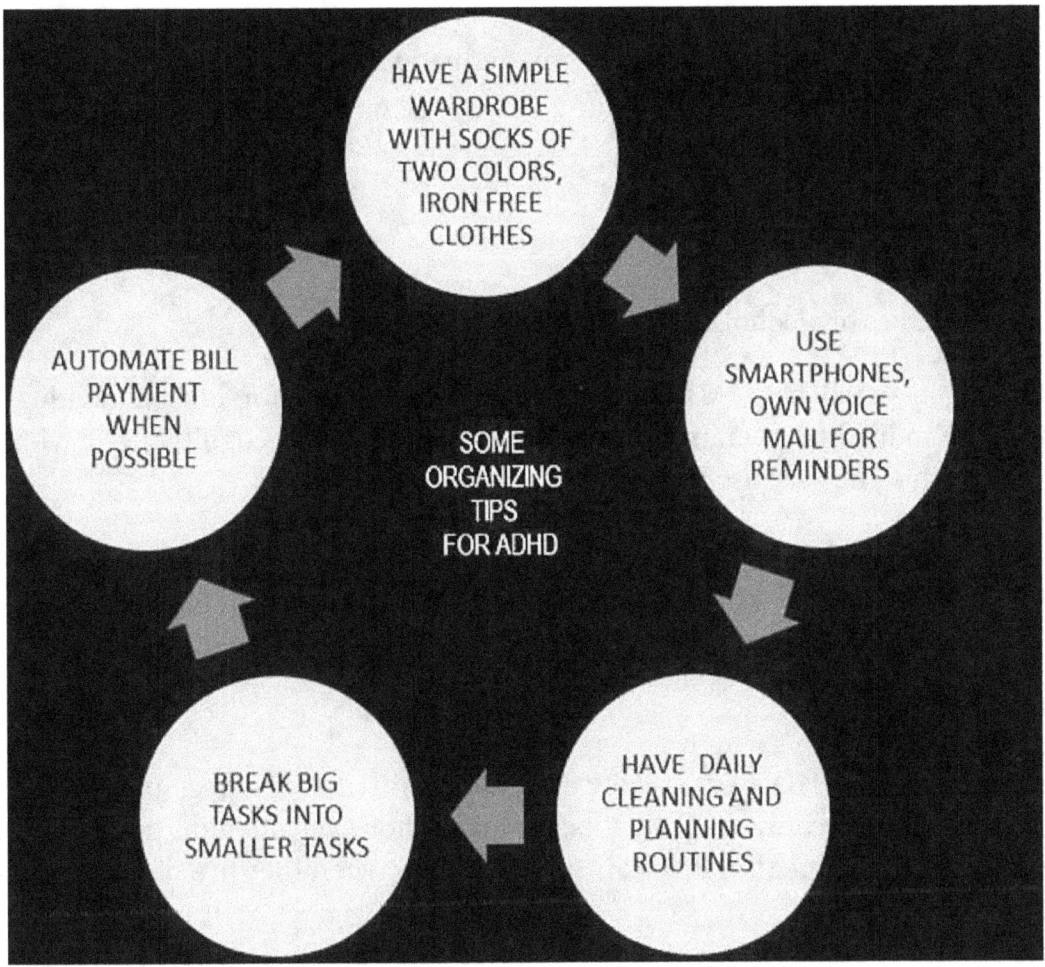

WHAT CAN I DO TO IMPROVE MY FUNCTIONING IF I HAVE ADHD?

The following tips may be useful in being more productive if the person has ADHD:

Have a regular time for organizing the home, office, and workspace.

Learn to use the calendar on your computer or smart phone and key in reminders, and alarms for important appointments.

Using post it notes is helpful for some individuals with ADHD. Get adequate amount of sleep and rest.

Eat a healthy and balanced diet.

Avoid conflict-laden relationships.

Avoid the use of alcohol or illicit substances.

Get professional help. Medications are relatively safe for most individuals. Getting individual therapy for emotional support and cognitive behavioral training may be very useful.

An ADHD coach can be very supportive resource that will help you stay on task with your goals and projects.

HOW LONG DOES IT TAKE TO ADJUST TO THE NON-ADHD LIFESTYLE?

At first, the ADHD patient may be giddy with the prospect of unlimited success when treatment is first begun. This however should be tempered with the knowledge that they can still have days when they are distracted due to other factors.

It may take a while for the person to adjust to a normal ADHD free lifestyle. It is important to not become overzealous in correcting every behavior that they feel is related to ADHD.

Normalization means allowing for the occasional disorganization or forgetfulness. It is also important for the individual to recognize that their ADHD is not necessarily a liability in all situations. They may have bursts of creativity at times and they should be allowed to pursue their interests and vocations with the understanding that they may need to have assistance and help in wrapping things up and following through on their projects.

Remember that anyone can be taught to improve their time management and organizational skills. Thus, they can become more organized in the planning and less impulsive in their actions. This can in turn lead to lasting changes with resulting improvement in their interpersonal and professional lives.

In unusual circumstances, as is seen in some family members of alcohol dependent patients, a codependency issues might need to be addressed. The spouse or family member may offer some resistance as they may be used to the old impulsive fly by the seat partner that they had grown to love and care for.

They may thus consciously or unconsciously try to prevent their recovery to better patterns of relating and living. This family member or spouse may have their own issues that make them attractive to the dysfunctional individual. They may need to have counseling for themselves in order for them to not interfere in the recovery efforts of the person with ADHD.

The patient and the family should be educated that change will be gradual and subtle at first. Over time however, the increased productivity will become evident. It is important to acknowledge all progress made and provide positive feedback to the person with ADHD.

In the final analysis, it is important to remember that some days will be better than others. Sometime it's okay to go off the beaten track and allow free reign to their spirits and their daydreams. Some dreams can become wonderful realities. It is more important to recognize that they now have control over the organized and disorganized part of their lives and have the ability to change it for the better when they want to.

ADHD IN PRISON POPULATIONS

Studies have indicated that up to 25 percent of the imprisoned populations may have problems with ADHD. Given these numbers, the rehabilitation plans for these individuals must include an assessment for ADHD so that proper treatment and rehabilitation can be planned. Inmate rehabilitation is more likely to succeed if ADHD is treated when it exists. With treatment, impulsivity is decreased allowing for greater discretion and better judgment on the part of the individual in the future.

Treatment of ADHD can give the individual with ADHD just enough brakes to consider the consequences before they commit their next crime.

A willful disregard of validated incidence of ADHD and not offering treatment to affected prisoners may be shortsighted and negligent. Treatment with non-stimulants can be cheap while incarceration of these individuals in prisons on a revolving door basis is much more expensive. Aside from decreasing crime and incarceration, treatment of individuals in prison is the humane thing to do and will go towards making us a better society.

One of the obstacles to treating ADHD has been its automatic association with stimulant medications that can lend themselves to abuse. A rational plan should involve treatments that do not involve the use of stimulants but resort to other non-medication options that have also proven a remarkable efficacy in treating this condition.

One of these medications that was approved in the last decade is Guanfacine. It is also marketed under the brand name Intuniv. The reason that some consumers might balk at the use of Intuniv is its price. This problem however can be overcome by using the generic guanfacine which has a long half-life of almost 17 hours and can be used in a once a day or twice a day regimen for the control of ADHD symptoms.

The topic of ADHD in the prison populations is an area that has not been fully explored, and in due time, more data will be available. In general, it is fair to say that the treatment of ADHD in the prison populations is often neglected and overlooked. This fact provides the administrators and clinicians an opportunity to improve the rehabilitation of these individuals. Treatment can lessen the financial and social burden of incarceration and everything associated with it.

With treatment, there is a real chance of avoiding the initial incarceration and incarceration through recidivism. Locking someone away is some deterrent against crime but it will not change the underlying neurobiology of ADHD. If any correctional system is honestly invested in rehabilitating the citizen, then they must look at the problem of addressing untreated mental illness including the illness of ADHD.

Those with a prior history of substance or alcohol use problems should not be prescribed stimulant medications that can be diverted, or misused in further criminal enterprises.

The most beneficial interventions are as follows

1. Treatment of ADHD with nonstimulant medications

2. Teaching of TM and other meditations in prisons and jails

3. Neurofeedback treatment of ADHD

4. Teaching of organizational skills and healthy lifestyles

5. Vocational and job training that is suitable for ADHD

When treatment of ADHD is provided through rehabilitation, a better outcome is likely.

 It is likely to lower the rates of recidivism and of future criminal activity.

It also allows an opportunity for individual to make a contribution to society in productive ways rather than being a burden through incarceration.

Chapter 8
Resources & Further Reading

Resources on the Internet

1. www.chadd.org This is a good site for children and adults with ADHD

2. Attention! Magazine www.chadd.org

3. ADDitude Magazine www.chadd.org

4. ADD Consults www.addconsults.com

What are some organizations that can be a resource for further information and guidance?

NAMI [the national alliance on mental illness]

They have local chapters and also are on the internet at

www.nami.org

This is a unique website for ADHD Coaching

www.ADHDcoaches.org

The website can provide telephone number of a local ADHD coach that guides the person with different life issues touched by ADHD. It may be affordable for many and is worth looking into.

National Institute of Mental Health (NIMH)

This a national organization that promotes research and education on areas related to mental health. They have informative brochures and listing of other resources. The website address is

www.nimh.nih.gov

ADDA (Attention Deficit Disorder Association) This is an association that advocates for those with ADHD. Their contact information as follows:

- Tel 1888-638-3999

- Email: www.adda.org

CHADD (Children and Adults with ADHD) is a similar organization.

Additude Magazine: this is a free weekly newsletter that addresses routine problems of ADHD adults and children. It often has useful advice

Office of civil rights at the US Department of Education may also be able to provide support and information about section 504 of the rehabilitation act

ADHD's support groups.

These can be located at the following website www.chadd.org

Other Sources of Support

- Local Community Mental Health Center

- Local TM Teacher Tel 1888-LEARN-TM

- TM on the internet at www.tm.org

OTHER BOOKS ON ADHD THAT MAY BE HELPFUL

1. Driven To Distraction by John Ratey MD, Edward Hallowell MD

2. Making the System Work for Your Child with ADHD by Peter S. Jensen MD

3. The ADHD Workbook for Parents: A Guide for Parents of Children Ages 2-12 with Attention-Deficit/Hyperactivity Disorder by Harvey C Parker PhD

4. Life at Full Throttle: Attention Deficit/Hyperactivity Disorder in Adults by Catherine Avery

5. Women with Attention Deficit Disorder: Embrace Your Differences and Transform Your Life by Sari Solden

6. You Mean I'm Not Lazy, Stupid or Crazy?!: A Self-Help Book for Adults with Attention Deficit Disorder by Kate Kelly

7. Taking Charge of ADHD: The Complete, Authoritative Guide for Parents by Russell A. Barkley

8. Is It You, Me, or Adult ADD? Stopping the Roller Coaster When Someone You Love Has Attention Deficit Disorder By Gina Pera

9. Among the Jimson Weeds (Running Nowhere, By Paul Keene

10. 365 Ways to Succeed With Adhd: A Full Year Of Valuable Tips And Strategies From The World's Best Coaches And Experts (Volume 1) By Laurie D. Dupar

11. 10 ADD Friendly ways to organize your life by Judith Kohlberg

12. ADD and the College Student: A Guide for High School and College Students with Attention Deficit Disorder by Patricia O. Quinn, MD

WHAT IS THE AMERICANS WITH DISABILITIES (ADA) ACT?

The ADA is a civil rights law that bans and prohibits any discrimination based on disability. It is similar to the Civil Rights Act of 1964, which made discrimination based on race, religion, sex, or country of origin, and other characteristics illegal. Disability is defined by the ADA as "...a physical or mental impairment that substantially limits a major life activity." The determination of disability is made on a case-by-case basis.

This act requires educational institutions to make accommodations under Section 504 of 1973 Americans with Disabilities Act. They are mandated to make academic accommodation for individuals with disabilities in order to optimize the career and educational potential of their courses.

WHAT KIND OF ASSISTANCE ON THE JOB MIGHT BE AVAILABLE FOR PERSONS WITH ADHD?

People with ADHD may be able to boost their performance in the workplace through job coaching or mentoring. The mentor will help with organization skills, such as taking notes, keeping a daily planner and prioritizing a to-do list. Patients may do better in a quiet workspace with few distractions. ADHD is a disability under the Americans with Disabilities Act. This means employers must make adjustments to support a worker's needs.

WHAT IS SECTION 504 AND IEP?

This section of the law requires institutions of learning to provide special accommodations for individuals with disabilities that may interfere with learning. The disability may be physical or psychological in nature.

Some accommodations of section 504 for individuals with ADHD may be the following:

- The availability of a quiet area with decreased distractions

- Decreased workload for homework

- Providing extra time for tests

- Use of organizers and notebooks for communication between parents and teachers may be encouraged.

- Use of recording device such as a tape recorder may be allowed

An IEP or individualized educational plan is a special plan developed keeping in mind the specific deficits of the child. It sets specific goals for the child and may use behavioral management techniques such as a reward system to encourage the achievement of goals.

Chapter 9
Epilogue

We have taken a journey together looking into the diagnosis of ADHD, and its myriad manifestations. We have also taken a look into ways to overcome the difficulties.

Knowledge as they say is power. If you are a person with ADHD, this is powerful and useful information that you now possess. It can be used for improving the quality of your life and to help you gain the level of success that you deserve.

If you are a clinician, it has hopefully provided you with a conviction that ADHD can be treated and that such patients should be offered an eclectic choice of treatment options. It does not have to necessarily be medications but they are an important tool in many cases of ADHD. The clinician should not shy away from offering treatment. The treatment of ADHD can be professionally gratifying for the clinician and the patient. Many of the treatments have a proven track record of good safety profile and efficacy. The results are noticeable and achieved over a relatively short period of time.

If you are a family member, your new found knowledge may allow you to appreciate the difficulties that ADHD can cause. This may allow you to take a more patient and compassionate approach when interacting with a family member that has ADHD.

Looking towards the future, progress in finding newer medications for ADHD is possible. One always need to temper the hope for a magic pill with the understanding that ADHD is multifaceted condition that will require a concerted biopsychosocial approach over time for the best results. It will always be a collaborative effort involving education, medications, meditation, psychotherapy, and interventions unique to the person's situation. The clinician with an open approach to different ideas is always more helpful to his patients than the clinician with a single tool for treatment.

Some prospects for new medications include other norepinephrine or dopamine reuptake inhibitors or medications that affect the cholinergic system.

Neurofeedback should be developed further and the technology may become more affordable. This may revolutionize the treatment of ADHD by even removing the stigma of taking stimulant meds and attendant worries of addiction, diversion or side effects.

It is possible that our knowledge about the genetics of ADHD will increase. This will allow labs in the future perhaps to map the full human genome with relatively little cost. We may be able to choose a particular medication for a certain subset of diseases such as hypertension, diabetes, ADHD or others based on the particular genetics or genotype that is more responsive to a specific class of medications.

Genetic research may yield more detailed information about the genetics of inheritance. The interaction of subtle changes in the genotype and environment is a vast area. There are likely to be multiple genes encoding for different receptors and enzymes that will be implicated.

We must cherish however the uniqueness of our individuals with ADHD. They are not mistakes necessarily of development. God works in mysterious ways and provides each human being with a genome slightly different from every living thing that has existed or will exist. This difference can be a gift or a liability depending on the circumstance. This perhaps is the reason that the label of an illness on a multifaceted illness such as ADHD is hard to impose and hard to accept at times.

Individuals with ADHD are unique people that can learn to complement their natural out of the box thinking with methods to become more organized and focused. With the help of options discussed in this book, they are uniquely positioned to achieve the goals that may have eluded them.

The success they find may surprise the person with ADHD and others. Many of the interventions are relatively safe and the potential benefits are significant.

It is fair to say that there is much hope for individuals that have ADHD and ADD. With treatment, they can still realize and actualize all that their potential carries and may be something extra that no one else has!

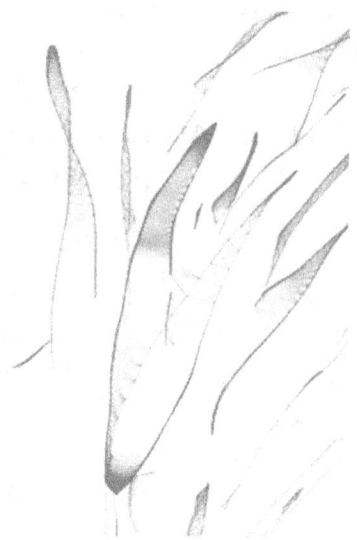

"The human spirit is never finished when it is defeated... it is finished when it surrenders." Ben Stein

Other Books by the Author

Overcoming Anxiety

A Single Idea Can Make a Difference

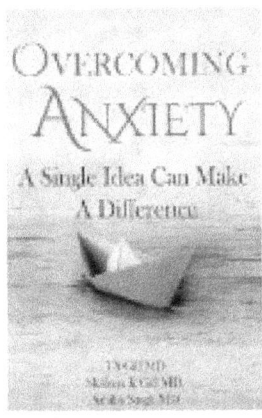

http://www.amazon.com/Overcoming-Anxiety-Single-Idea-Difference/ d p/09 896 649 29/ref=sr _ 1 _ 1 ?ie=UTF8&qid= 141 26599 70& sr=8-1&keywords=tirath+s+gill+MD

HANDBOOK OF EMERGENCY PSYCHIATRY

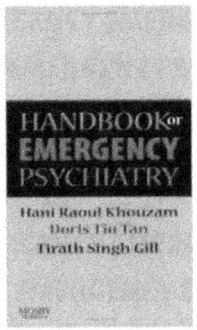

http://www.amazon.com/Handbook-Emergency-Psychiatry-Hani-Khouzam/dp/0323040888/ref=sr_1_1?ie=UTF8&qid=1399880616&sr=8-1&keywords=Tirath+s+gill+md

HOW TO ACHIEVE YOUR GOALS:
LEADERSHIP LESSONS FROM ALEXANDER THE GREAT

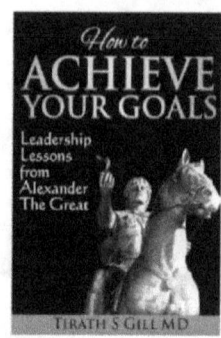

http://www.amazon.com/How-Achieve-Your-Goals-Leadership/
dp/0989664902/ref=sr_1_fkmr1_1?ie=UTF8&qid=1399880826&sr=8-1-fk
mr1&keywords=Tirath+s+gill+md